Immune Boosting Cookbook

Healthy Immune Can Help You Fighting Several Diseases

BY

Stephanie Sharp

License Notes

Table of Contents

Introduction

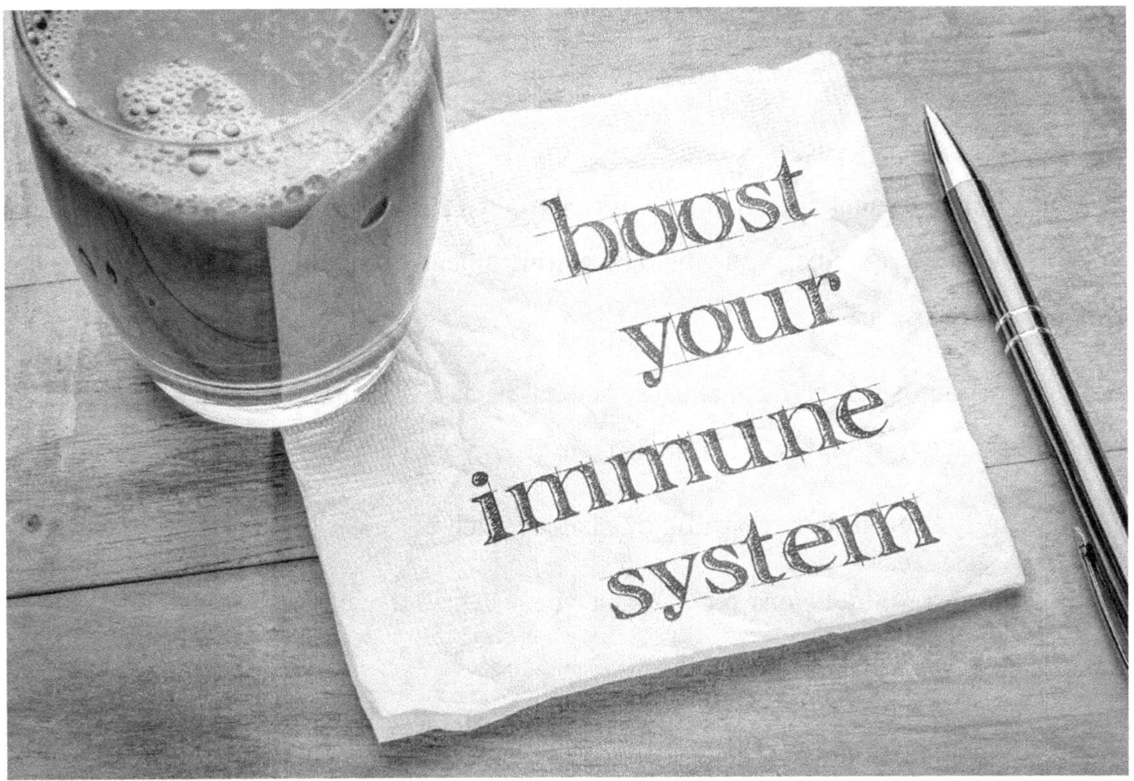

Chances for people with a low immune system are very high to experience several health conditions such as high fever, vomit, stomachache and a lot more. They often get sick even with a slight climate change.

I have seen a lot of individuals who often take medicines for small allergies like mild fever, cold or cough. Please understand that taking medicines for everything would not help you boost your immune system. You are rather making your body's natural defense system to depend upon the medicines.

Consuming healthy recipes, exposure to sunlight, plenty of water intake, walking and a minimum of 8 hours of sleep are all considered to be the keys which can help you get a healthy immune system.

Remember, you are actually in charge of your own body's defense system and need to take effective steps for it.

A diet that includes junk food & plenty of sugar may have adverse effects on your immune system. With the right diet, you would be getting a healthy immune and numerous health benefits too. These are:

-   To fight pathogens (germs that cause several diseases) such as viruses, bacteria, fungi or parasites, and to completely eliminate them from your body

-   To identify & neutralizing harmful substances (such as cancer cells) present in the body.

This e-book has 45 delicious recipes that you can try at your home (includes healthy smoothies, breakfast, lunch, dinner & soups).

Healthy Smoothies

Strawberry Kiwi Smoothie

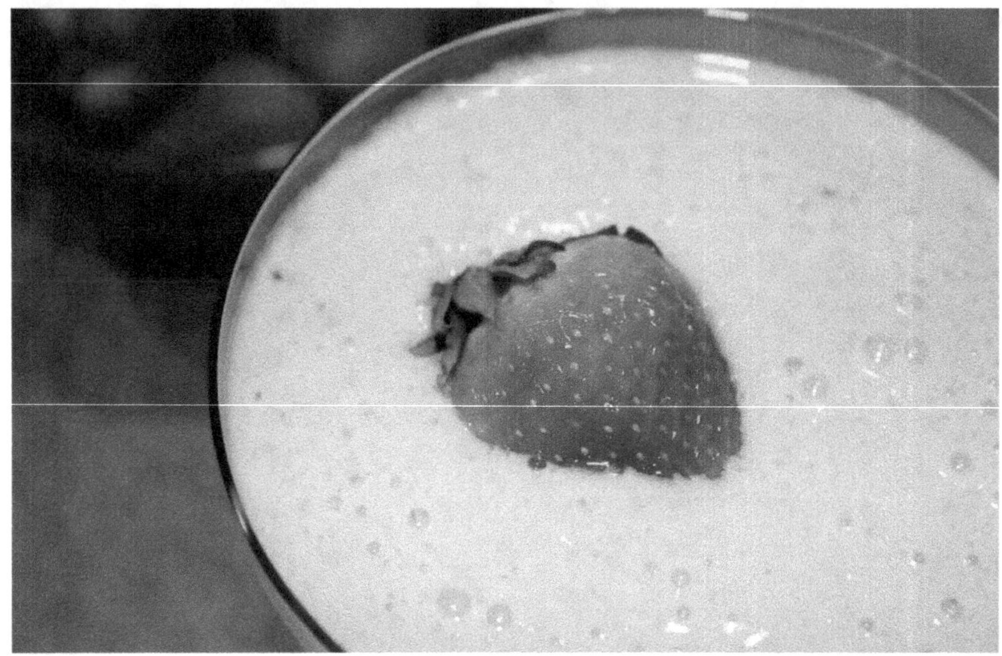

Prep Time: 2 minutes

Cooking Time: 3 minutes

Servings: 2 persons

It tastes amazing and quite a refreshing drink to kick-start your day with. You can enjoy this drink on a hot sunny day. Feel free to sub frozen vanilla yogurt with frozen non-dairy ice cream.

Ingredients:

- ½ cup frozen vanilla yogurt
- 6 strawberries, hulled & coarsely chopped
- ½ banana, partially frozen
- 1 kiwi, peeled & coarsely chopped
- ½ cup each of orange juice & pineapple juice
- Ice cubes

Directions:

1. Combine the entire ingredients together in a blender. Blend on high power until completely smooth & creamy, for a minute.

2. Serve immediately & enjoy.

Nutritional Value: kcal: 174, Fat: 1.3 g, Fiber: 3 g, Protein: 5 g, Carbohydrates: 38 g

Carrot & Ginger Smoothie

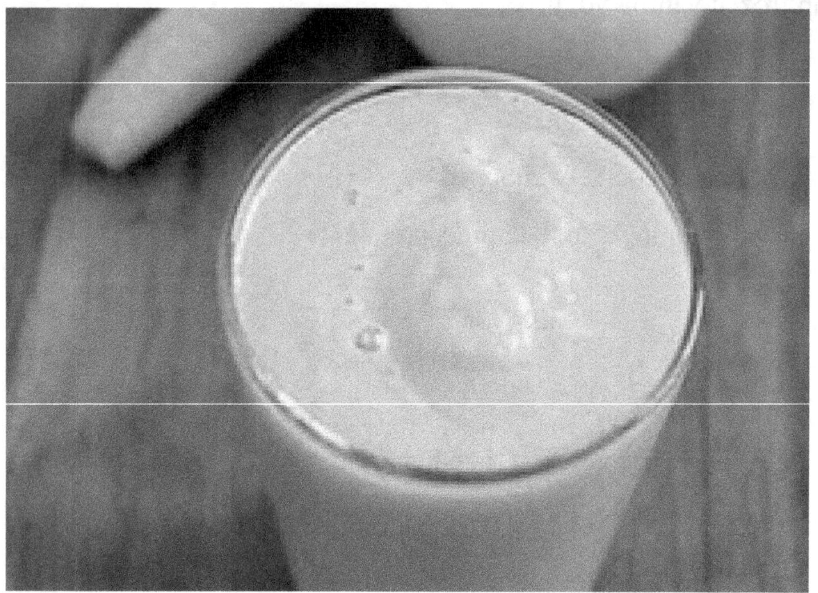

Prep Time: 2 minutes

Cooking Time: 2 minutes

Servings: 2 persons

This healing drink is good for your digestive track. You would forget about your morning coffee or tea after you try this at your home.

Ingredients:

- 1 apple, unpeeled, cored & quartered
- 4 unpeeled carrots
- 1 stalk celery, fresh, preferably with leaves
- 1 ounce piece of ginger, peeled (approximately a thumb size)

Directions:

1. Put the entire ingredients together in a magic bullet or blender. Blend on high power until completely smooth.

2. Serve immediately & enjoy.

Nutritional Value: kcal: 112, Fat: 1 g, Fiber: 6 g, Protein: 1.7 g, Carbohydrates: 27 g

Berry Kale Ginger Smoothie

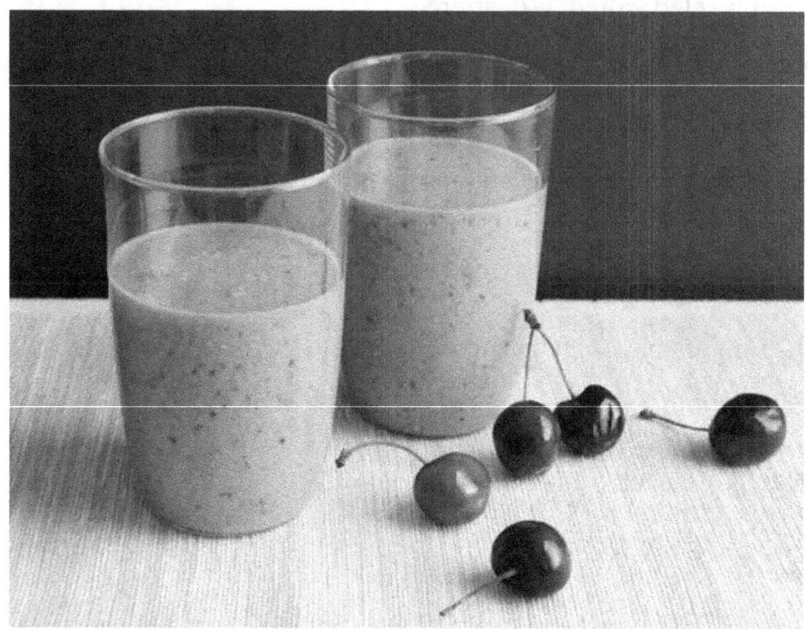

Prep Time: 2 minutes

Cooking Time: 2 minutes

Servings: 1 person

Ginger and kale have a lot of health benefits, and you would fall in love with the taste. To improve the taste, you can even add a teaspoon of raw honey to it. Absolutely amazing!

Ingredients:

- ½" ginger
- 1 cup kale, tightly packed
- 6 berries, frozen
- 1 tablespoon lemon juice, freshly squeezed
- 6 almonds
- 1 medium banana
- 2 cups water

Directions:

1. Add kale in a medium-sized measuring cup then, add a splash of lemon juice followed by ginger, berries and almonds. Fill the cup with water and blend at high speed in a Vitamix.

2. Add banana & continue to blend until blended well at medium speed. Pour the mixture into a large glass; serve immediately & enjoy.

Nutritional Value: kcal: 162, Fat: 4.6 g, Fiber: 4 g, Protein: 4 g, Carbohydrates: 31 g

Healthy Broccoli Smoothie

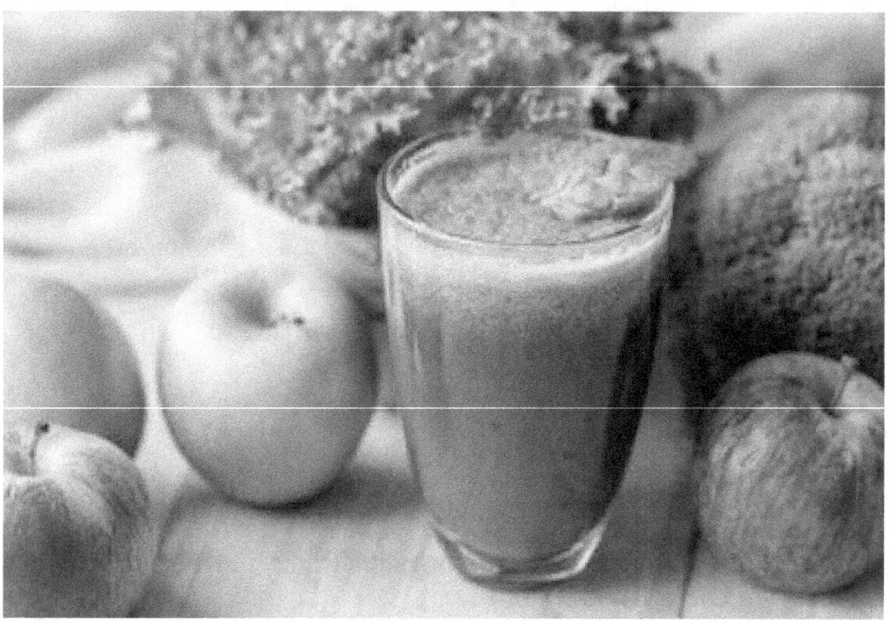

Prep Time: 2 minutes

Cooking Time: 2 minutes

Servings: 2 persons

Have you ever imagined that you could even use broccoli in a drink too? This smoothie has greenhouse effect and has essential vitamins, fiber and minerals but very low in overall calories. While blending, feel free to add a tablespoon of turbinado sugar to the drink.

Ingredients:

- 4 broccoli florets, chopped
- 1 carrot, chopped
- 2 cups fresh spinach leaves
- 1 cup orange juice, to dilute
- 2 mandarin orange sections
- Ice Cubes

Directions:

1. Combine the entire ingredients together in a blender. Blend on high power until completely smooth & creamy.

2. Serve immediately and enjoy.

Nutritional Value: kcal: 240, Fat: 2 g, Fiber: 10 g, Protein: 9 g, Carbohydrates: 36 g

Berry Banana Yogurt Smoothie

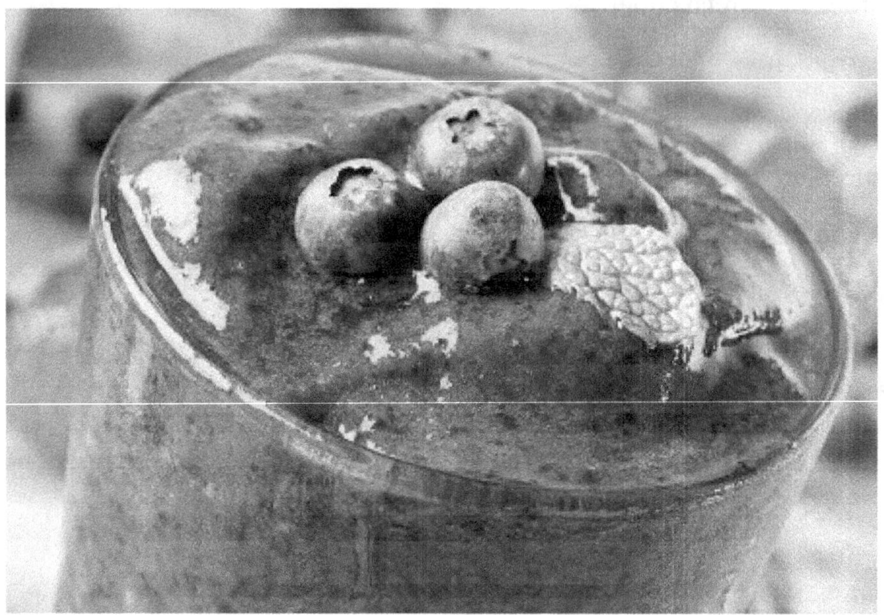

Prep Time: 2 minutes

Cooking Time: 2 minutes

Servings: 1 person

Absolutely delicious & quite easy to prepare! Each ingredient mentioned in the smoothie is good for your stomach. A healthy stomach means a healthy immune. You can certainly garnish your drink with a strawberry and sprinkle few nuts on top.

Ingredients:

- ½ cup cranberries
- 1 cup cold chamomile tea
- ½ papaya
- 1 cup Greek yoghurt
- ½ banana, frozen
- ½ cup blueberries

Directions:

1. Combine the entire ingredients together in a blender. Blend on high power until completely smooth & creamy.

2. Serve immediately and enjoy.

Nutritional Value: kcal: 295, Fat: 4.2 g, Fiber: 6 g, Protein: 14 g, Carbohydrates: 32 g

Lime Papaya Mango Smoothie

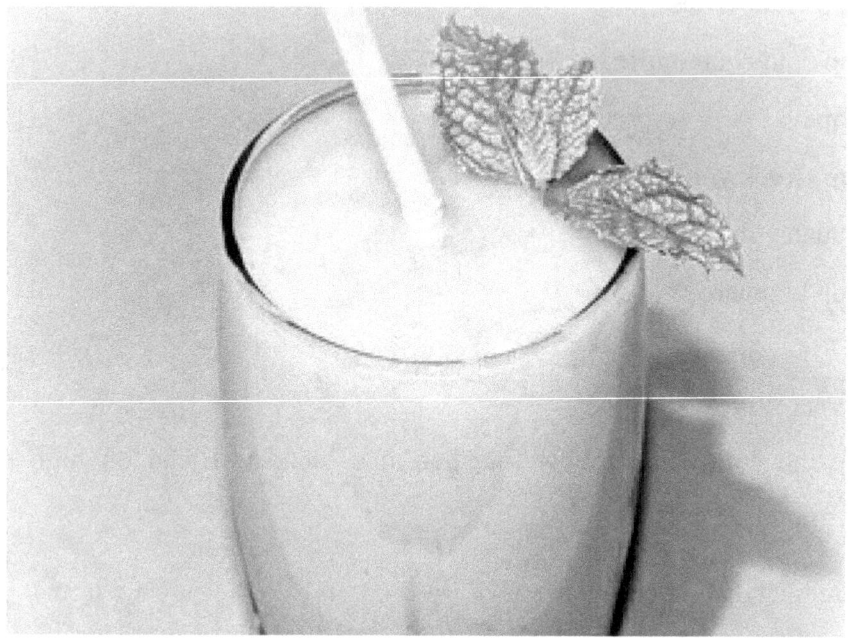

Prep Time: 2 minutes

Cooking Time: 2 minutes

Servings: 2 persons

You can always try this healthy smoothie early in the morning. You can garnish your drink with a lime slice and fresh mint. Enjoy the taste!

Ingredients:

- ½ cup mango, peeled & chopped
- 1 cup nut milk
- 3 tablespoons lime juice, freshly squeezed
- ½ cup papaya, peeled & chopped
- 1 dash of vanilla extract, raw

Directions:

1. Combine the entire ingredients together in a blender. Blend on high power for a minute, until completely smooth & creamy.

2. Serve immediately and enjoy.

Nutritional Value: kcal: 80, Fat: 1.5 g, Fiber: 2 g, Protein: 2 g, Carbohydrates: 10 g

Spinach Apple Smoothie

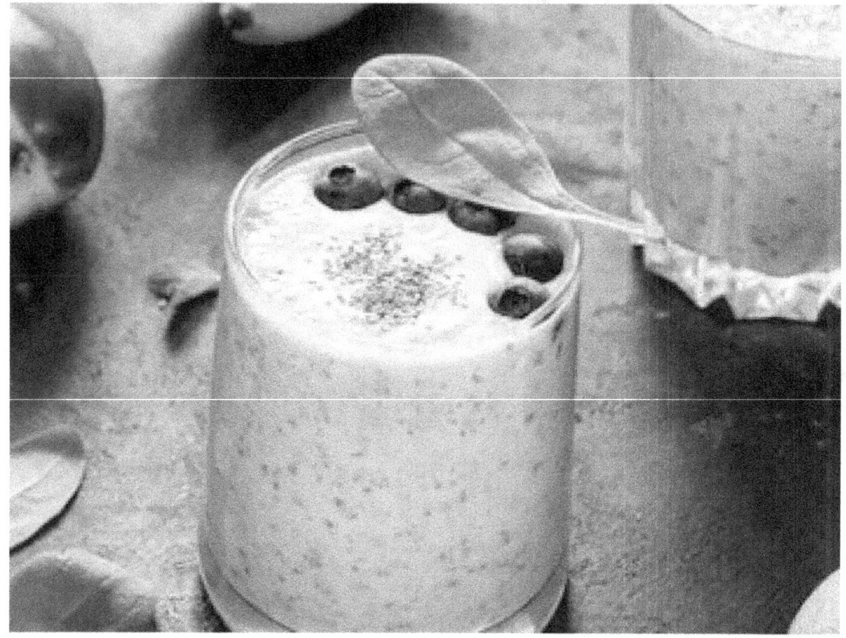

Prep Time: 2 minutes

Total Time: 2 minutes

Servings: 1

Absolutely refreshing and a healthy drink to kick-start your day!   You can even add a carrot and a tablespoon of raw honey.

Ingredients:

- 1 small apple, cut up into chunks
- ½ teaspoon cinnamon
- 1 small banana, frozen
- 2 cups fresh spinach
- 1 cup almond milk

Directions:

1. Combine the entire ingredients together in a blender. Blend on high power until completely smooth & creamy.

2. Serve immediately and enjoy.

Nutritional Value: kcal: 240, Fat: 3.3 g, Fiber: 8 g, Protein: 5 g, Carbohydrates: 36 g

Kale Orange & Watermelon Smoothie

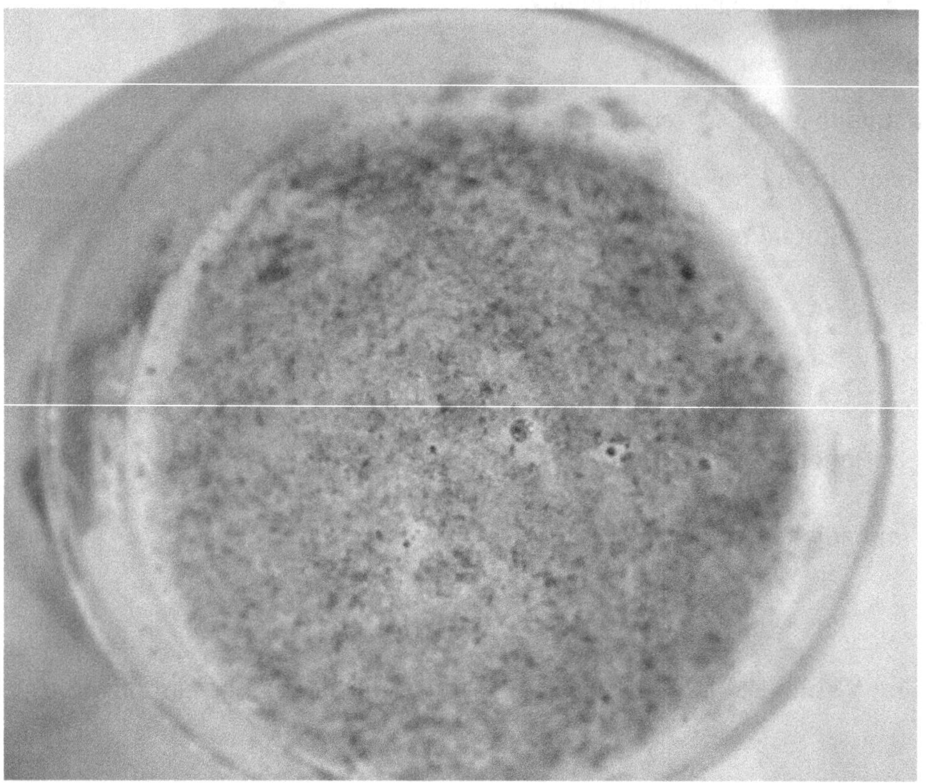

Prep Time: 2 minutes

Total Time: 5 minutes

Servings: 5 persons

My family just loved the taste, and I am glad that I prepared this healthy drink for them. You can skip ground flaxseed or coconut oil and can add a tablespoon or two of raw honey or turbinado sugar.

Ingredients:

- 1 cup fresh kale
- 3 large oranges
- ½ cup fresh spinach
- 1 lemon
- Fresh mint leaves, chopped
- ¼ whole watermelon
- 2 tablespoons coconut oil
- 1 tablespoon ground flax seeds

Directions:

1. Steam the spinach and kale over boiling water for 5 minutes; let cool.

2. Chop the entire ingredients and then, blend in a blender with some water, on high power until completely smooth and creamy. Serve and enjoy.

Nutritional Value: kcal: 122, Fat: 6.2 g, Fiber: 3.6 g, Protein: 2 g, Carbohydrates: 17 g

Dr.Oz's Green Drink

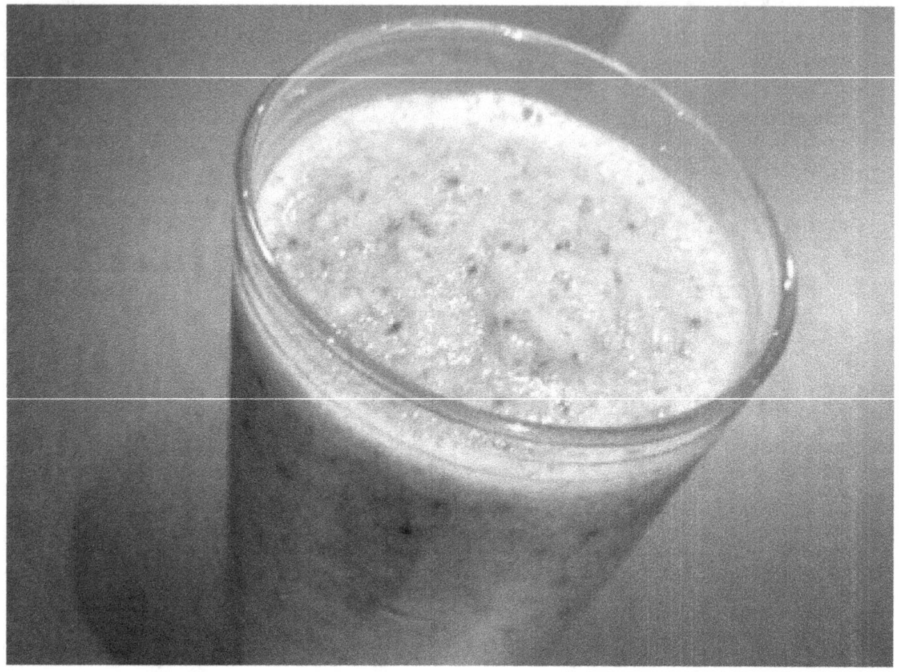

Prep Time: 5 minutes

Cooking Time: 5 minutes

Servings: 4 persons

If your smoothie appears to be too thick, then you can add water to it until you get your desired consistency. Likewise, you can adjust the amount of lime, lemon or sweetener to your likings. Feel free to garnish your drink with a cucumber slice and fresh cilantro leaves.

Ingredients:

- 2 cups spinach
- 1 celery stalk
- 1 -2 medium cucumber
- ½" gingerroot
- Juice of 1 lime, freshly squeezed
- 2 apples, cored
- 1 bunch fresh parsley, chopped
- 4 ounces mineral water or ice cubes
- Juice of ½ lemon, freshly squeezed

Optional Ingredients:

- Banana
- Unsweetened fruit juice
- Raw carrot

Directions:

1. Combine the entire ingredients together in a blender (along with any optional ingredient) & blend on high power for a minute, until completely smooth & creamy.

2. Serve immediately and enjoy.

Nutritional Value: kcal: 70, Fat: 0.5 g, Fiber: 3 g, Protein: 1.5 g, Carbohydrates: 15 g

Awesome Spinach Smoothie

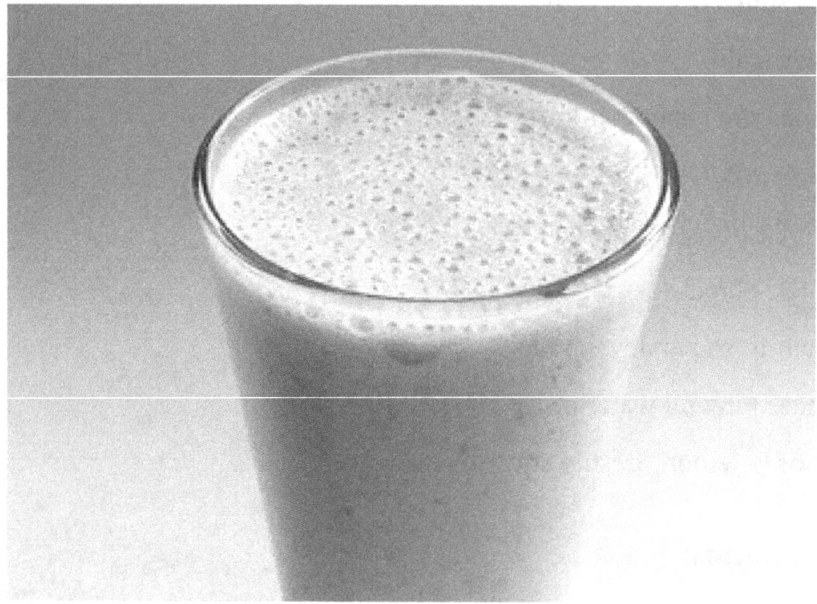

Prep Time: 5 minutes

Cooking Time: 5 minutes

Servings: 2 persons

The best part ever about this smoothie is that it would boost your immune system quickly, like anything. If the spinach and granny smith apple are too tart, the, feel free to add some sweetener or maple syrup to your taste. You can even create popsicles from the spinach smoothie as well. Enjoy.

Ingredients:

- 1 granny smith apple, peeled
- 8 ounces spinach
- 1 banana
- 1 orange, large, peeled
- 1 cup water or a handful of ice cubes

Directions:

1. Combine the entire ingredients together in a blender. Blend on high power until completely smooth & creamy.

2. Serve immediately and enjoy

Nutritional Value: kcal: 155, Fat: 1 g, Fiber: 7 g, Protein: 6 g, Carbohydrates: 20 g

Breakfast

Crunchy Spiced Chickpea Toast

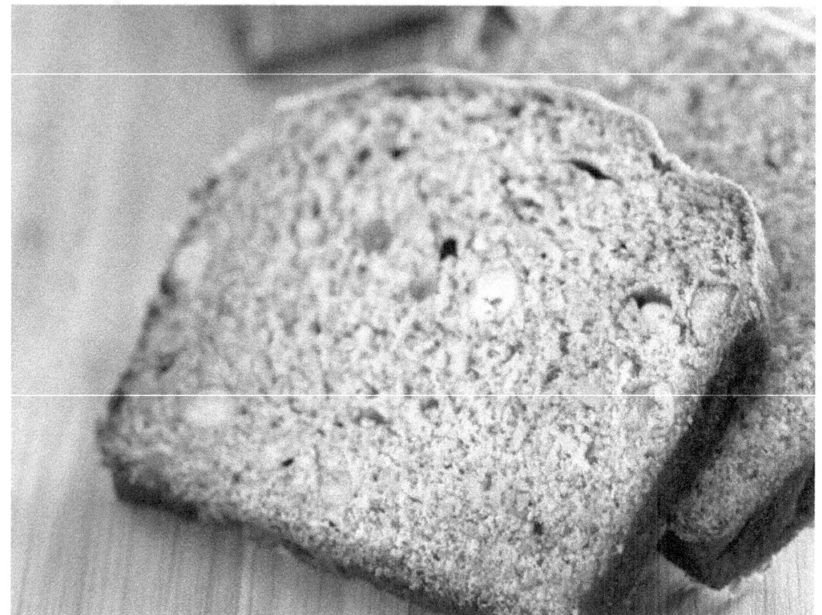

Prep Time: 5 minutes

Cooking Time: 10 minutes

Servings: 2 persons

This is surely one of the best toast recipes that I have ever prepared. This recipe includes whole grains, leafy greens and legumes. You can nourish your muscle growth with it and can get plenty of dietary fiber which is good for your heart health and digestion.

Ingredients:

- 2 slices whole wheat sourdough bread
- 1 avocado, ripe
- ¼ cup chickpeas, roasted
- 5 leaf mint leaves, fresh
- 1 tablespoon lemon zest
- ¼ teaspoon each of feta cheese, cayenne, ground ginger, ground cinnamon & salt

Directions:

1. Evenly spread the mashed avocado over the sourdough slices.

2. Next, toss the roasted chickpeas with cinnamon, ginger, cayenne & salt until mixed well.

3. Top the toast with the coated chickpeas.

4. Garnish with chopped mint leaves, feta cheese and fresh lemon zest. Serve immediately and enjoy.

Nutritional Value: kcal: 360, Fat: 13 g, Fiber: 11 g, Protein: 12 g, Carbohydrates: 35 g

Egg, Spinach and Portobello Breakfast Sandwich

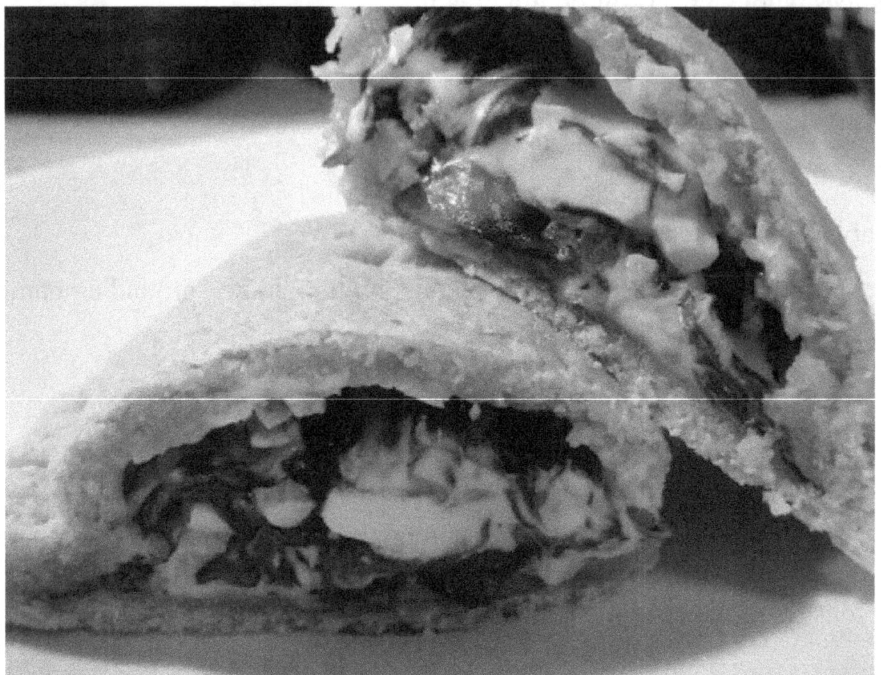

Prep Time: 15 minutes

Cooking Time: 10 minutes

Servings: 4 persons

Each muffin is spread with the goat cheese & stuffed with a mixture of Portobello mushrooms, eggs & baby spinach. You don't need any ketchup or anything with these sandwiches. Serve with your favorite fruit and enjoy the taste.

Ingredients:

- 4 English muffins, preferably whole-grain; fresh or toasted and cut into half
- 1 teaspoon lemon juice, fresh
- 3 oz goat cheese, soft
- ½ teaspoon ground black pepper
- 4 free-range eggs
- ¼ teaspoon sea salt
- 2 portabella mushroom caps
- 1 ½ teaspoons olive oil
- 4 oz baby spinach, fresh
- 1/8 teaspoon sea salt

Directions:

1. Evenly spread the goat cheese over each English muffin; set aside until ready to use.

2. Next, whisk the eggs together with fresh lemon juice, ¼ teaspoon of salt, and pepper in a medium-sized mixing bowl; set the mixture aside.

3. Next, over medium heat in a large, nonstick skillet; heat the oil until hot. Once done; add the spinach, mushrooms & sprinkle with the leftover salt; give the ingredients a good stir. Increase the heat to medium-high & sauté for 3 to 5 minutes, until the mushrooms are completely wilted & you don't find any excess liquid.

4. Decrease the heat to low and then, add the egg mixture; scramble softly for a minute or two. Transfer the cooked egg mixture to a large, clean bowl & set aside at room temperature for 3 to 5 minutes, until slightly cool. Strain any excess liquid off.

5. Now, add the prepared egg mixture over the English muffins and prepare the sandwiches. Serve and enjoy.

Nutritional Value: kcal: 269, Fat: 11 g, Fiber: 4 g, Protein: 16 g, Carbohydrates: 16 g

Peanut Butter Oatmeal Muffins

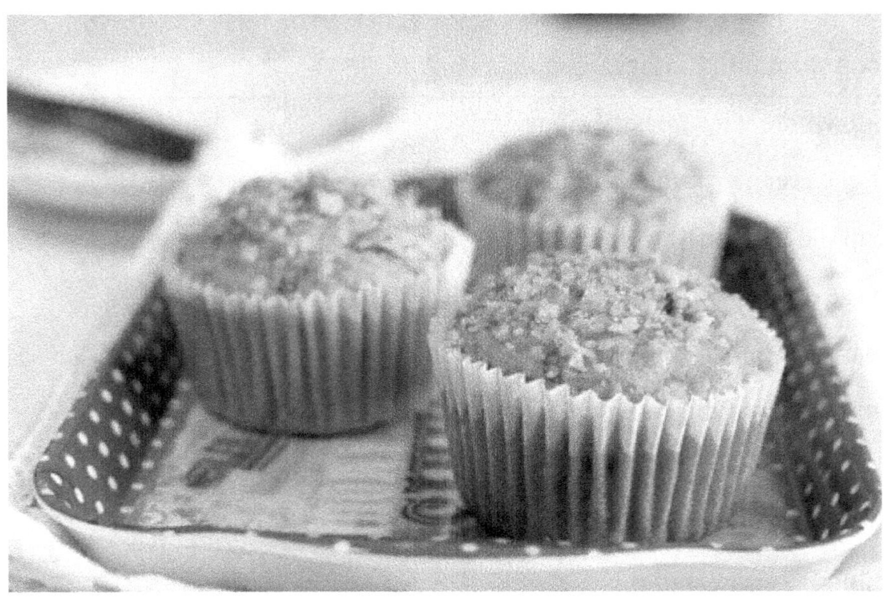

Prep Time: 20 minutes

Cooking Time: 20 minutes

Servings: 12 persons

The ingredients mentioned in this recipe are very easy to digest. The addition of blueberry jam makes this recipe a hit. You can even add raspberry jam or can use both i.e., blueberry jam and raspberry jam.

Ingredients:

- 1 ½ teaspoons baking powder
- ¾ cup skim milk, fat free
- 1 cup whole wheat pastry flour
- 1/3 cup creamy peanut butter
- 1 cup old fashioned rolled oats
- 2 large eggs, free-range
- 1 teaspoon pure vanilla extract
- ¾ teaspoon baking soda
- 1 1/8 cups turbinado cane sugar
- ¾ cup blueberry jam
- 2 tablespoons peanut oil
- ½ teaspoon sea salt

Directions:

1. Line a standard-sized muffin tray (with 12 cups) with muffin liners and then, preheat your oven to 425 F in advance.

2. Whisk the oats with baking soda, baking powder, flour, and salt in a medium-sized mixing bowl; set aside until ready to use.

3. Add peanut butter, peanut oil & milk to a blender; cover & puree on high power until completely smooth & creamy. Pour the batter into a large-sized mixing bowl.

4. Add eggs followed by the vanilla extract; continue to whisk until combined well. Add sugar & whisk until combined well.

5. Add the prepared oat mixture into the peanut butter mixture; give the ingredients a good stir for a minute or two, until just combined.

6. Evenly divide the batter among the prepared muffin cups (filling each cup approximately 7/8 full) and bake in your preheated oven for 15 to 20 minutes, until turn browned.

7. Let cool in the pan for a couple of minutes. Transfer the muffins to a wire rack. Then, let cool.

8. Once done; top each muffin with a tablespoon of the blueberry jam; serve immediately & enjoy.

Nutritional Value: kcal: 270, Fat: 7 g, Fiber: 3 g, Protein: 6 g, Carbohydrates: 40 g

Ham & Egg Cups

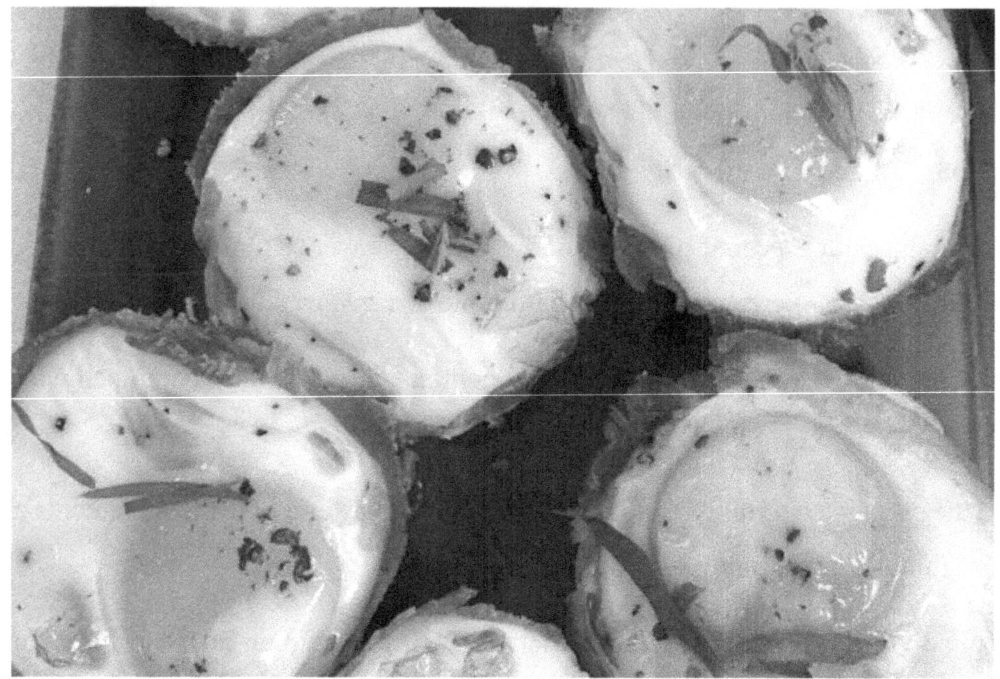

Prep Time: 30 minutes

Cooking Time: 35 minutes

Servings: 12 persons

This recipe is absolutely delicious, and I can guaranty you that you would prepare it often. For variety, you can flavor each cup with your favorite vegetables. Serve and enjoy.

Ingredients:

- 20 button mushrooms, medium
- 1 cup almond milk, unsweetened
- 26 slices applewood smoked ham, uncured
- 1 white onion, medium
- 12 whole egg, large
- 1 red bell pepper, medium
- 4 tablespoons olive oil
- 1/8 teaspoon each of black pepper, kosher salt & cayenne

Directions:

1. Preheat your oven to 425 F in advance.

2. Over medium heat in a large sauté pan; heat 2 tablespoons of oil until hot. Once done; swirl to coat the bottom of your pan completely. Next, add onions followed by peppers and mushrooms. Season with pepper and salt; cook until the moisture almost evaporates, for 8 to 10 minutes. Remove from the heat & reserve.

3. Lightly coat the inside of two muffin tins (preferably non-stick) with the remaining olive oil.

4. Press a slice of ham gently into each of the cups; forming a small bowl in each (ensure the ham is pressed against the sides but doesn't tear).

5. Chop the leftover slice of ham into very small bits; toss with the reserved peppers, onions and mushrooms.

6. Combine the eggs with almond milk, pepper, Cayenne and salt in a blender or with a whisk for a minute or two, until completely frothy.

7. Now, evenly fill the ham cups with the prepared egg mixture.

8. Put trays in the preheated oven & bake for 3 to 5 minutes.

9. Once done; remove & sprinkle the chopped mixture evenly into each cup.

10. Place the tray again into the oven & cook until the edges of the ham are crisp, for 7 to 10 minutes. Remove & serve. Enjoy.

Nutritional Value: kcal: 190, Fat: 11 g, Fiber: 0 g, Protein: 20 g, Carbohydrates: 3 g

Porridge with Blueberry Compote

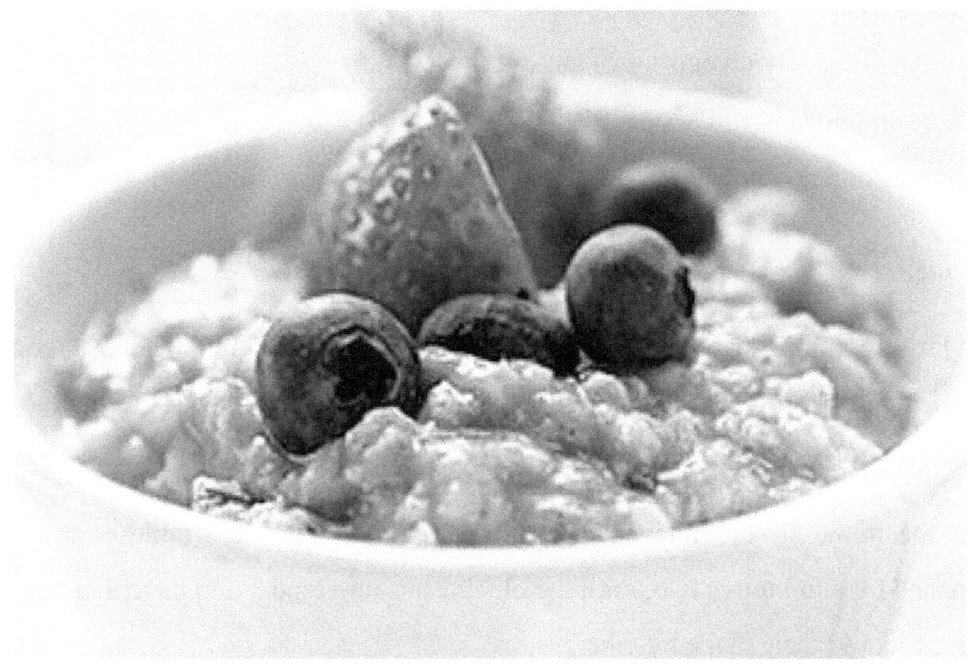

Prep Time: 5 minutes

Cooking Time: 5 minutes

Servings: 2 persons

This high-fiber delicious porridge is enough for your breakfast. You won't ask for anything else for your breakfast. The combination of oats and blueberries is well. You can top your dish with some dried coconut as well. You can even skip yoghurt and honey; if you use half water and half rice milk.

Ingredients:

- 1 cup blueberries, frozen

- 1 cup Greek-style yogurt, 0% fat

- 6 tablespoons porridge oats

- 1 teaspoon raw honey

Directions:

1. Fill a large, non-stick pan with approximately 3 cups of water; add the oats & cook until thickened, for 2 to 3 minutes, stirring occasionally, over moderate heat. Remove & 1/3 of your low-fat yogurt.

2. In the meantime, tip the blueberries into a pan with honey and 1 tablespoon of water; gently poach for a minute or two, until the blueberries turn tender and have thawed (ensure that they still hold their shape together).

3. Spoon the porridge into separate bowls and top each bowl with the leftover yogurt; spoon some blueberries on top. Serve immediately and enjoy.

Nutritional Value: kcal: 162, Fat: 3.3 g, Fiber: 2.4 g, Protein: 9 g, Carbohydrates: 26 g

Omelette pancakes with tomato & pepper sauce

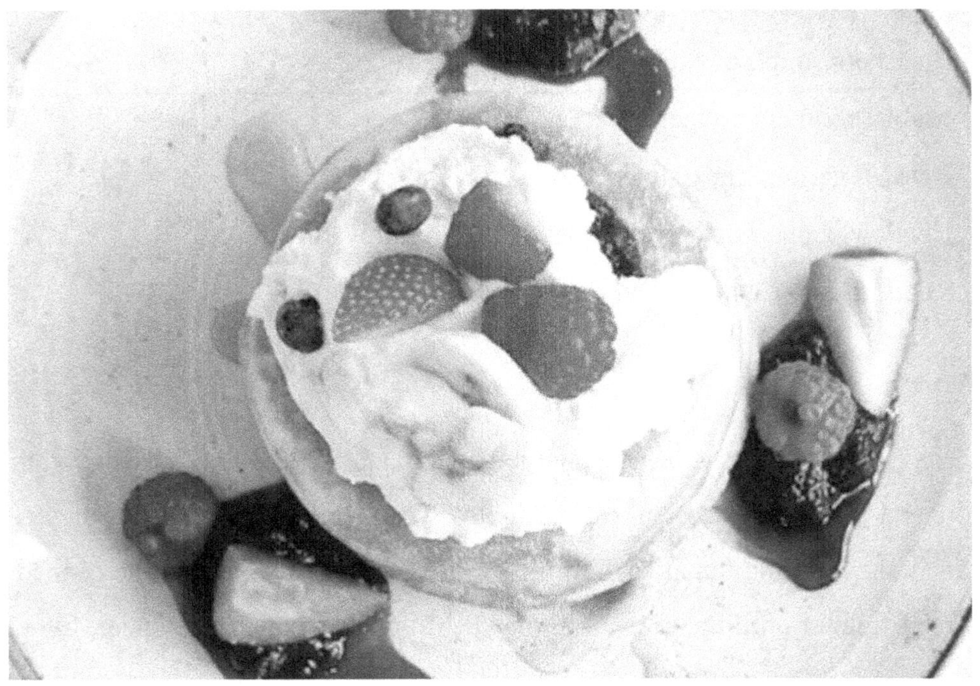

Prep Time: 10 minutes

Cooking Time: 20 minutes

Servings: 2 persons

For a quick breakfast meal, you can try this gluten-free and low-calorie recipe at your home. Believe me this recipe would become one of your favorites and you would prepare it often.

Ingredients:

- 4 organic eggs, large
- A handful of fresh basil leaves

For Sauce:

- 1 can chopped tomatoes (approximately 1 pound)
- 2 teaspoons rapeseed oil, plus more for the pancakes
- 1 tablespoon cider vinegar
- 2 cloves garlic, thinly sliced
- 1 yellow pepper, quartered, deseeded, then thinly sliced
- Salad leaves or whole-meal bread, to serve

Directions:

1. For Sauce: Over moderate heat in a large frying pan; heat the oil until hot and then, fry the garlic and pepper until soften, for 5 minutes. Then, spoon in the cider vinegar & let it sizzle away then, tip the tomatoes into the mixture followed by 1/3 of the canned water. Cover & let simmer until the sauce is somewhat thick & peppers are tender, for 12 to 15 minutes.

2. In the meantime, prepare the pancakes. Then, beat an egg with 1 teaspoon of water & seasoning. Next, coat a non-stick frying pan, preferably small sized with a small quantity of oil and heat it over moderate heat. Once hot; add the prepared egg mixture & cook until set into a thin pancake, for a minute or two. Carefully lift over a large plate; cover with aluminum foil & repeat the process with the remaining eggs. Roll up onto the warm plates and spoon some sauce on top; scatter with fresh basil. Lastly, serve with a fresh salad or bread on side and enjoy.

Nutritional Value: kcal: 271, Fat: 17 g, Fiber: 4 g, Protein: 16 g, Carbohydrates: 11 g

Greek Muffin-Tin Omelets with Feta & Peppers

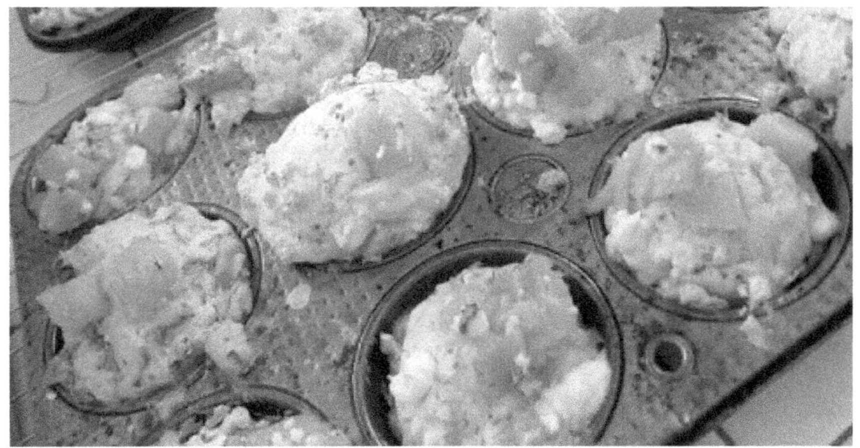

Prep Time: 20 minutes

Cooking Time: 30 minutes

Servings: 6 persons

These muffins are quite easy to prepare and taste great too. Just before serving, I sprinkled with some chili flakes and dried oregano. My entire family just loved it and asked me to make it again for them.

Ingredients:

- ¾ cup feta cheese, crumbled
- 1 red bell pepper, medium, diced
- ¾ cup onion, diced
- 2 cups fresh spinach, chopped
- ½ cup milk, low-fat
- 8 large eggs
- ½ teaspoon ground pepper
- 1 tablespoon fresh oregano, finely chopped
- ¼ cup Kalamata olives, sliced
- 2 tablespoons extra-virgin olive oil
- ¼ teaspoon salt, divided

Directions:

1. Generously coat a muffin tin (with 12 cups) with some cooking spray and then, preheat your oven to 325 F in advance.

2. Next, over medium heat in a large skillet; heat the oil until hot. Once done; add the onion & sprinkle with approximately 1/8 teaspoon of the salt; give the ingredients a good stir and cook for 2 to 3 minutes, until beginning to turn soften, stirring frequently. Add the bell pepper & oregano; continue to cook for 3 to 5 more minutes, until the vegetables have started to turn brown and are tender, stirring frequently. Remove from the heat; set aside and let cool for a couple of minutes.

3. Now, in a large bowl; whisk eggs with milk, feta, pepper and the leftover salt until mixed well. Stir in the olives, spinach and the prepared vegetable mixture. Evenly divide the mixture among the coated muffin cups.

4. Bake in the preheated oven for 20 to 25 minutes, until firm to the touch. Let stand for a couple of minutes. Then, remove the muffins from the tin. Serve warm and enjoy.

Nutritional Value: kcal: 220, Fat: 17 g, Fiber: 1.5 g, Protein: 13 g, Carbohydrates: 6 g

Savory Oatmeal with Cheddar, Collards & Eggs

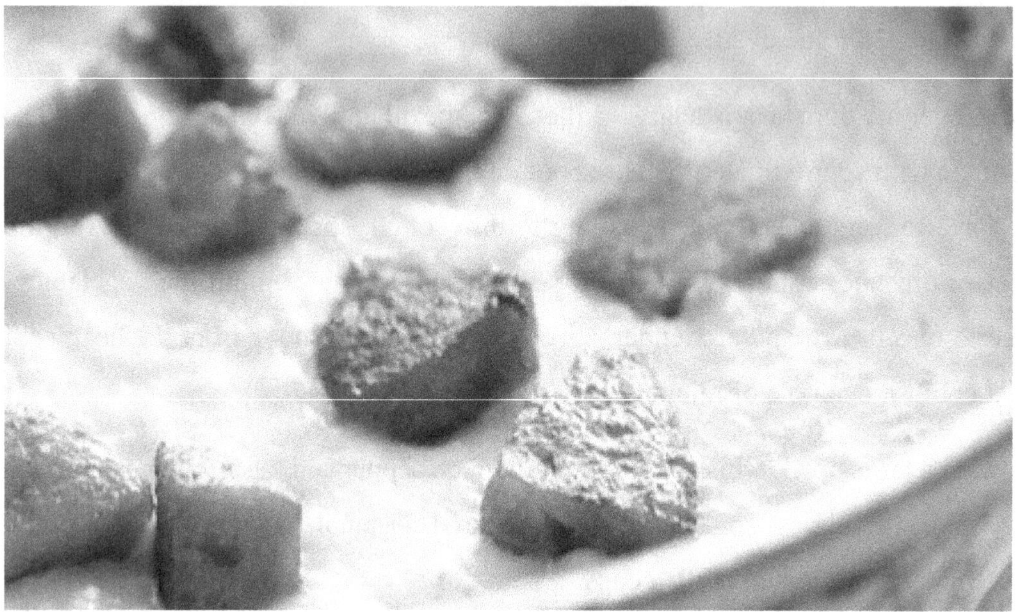

Prep Time: 30 minutes

Cooking Time: 30 minutes

Servings: 4 persons

Ensure that you use gluten-free oats for this recipe. For added protein, I added a hard-boiled egg on top along with some collards and even more of salsa. Taste great and quite easy to prepare!

Ingredients:

- 2 tablespoons shallot, diced
- 10 cups collard greens, chopped
- 4 cups plus ½ cup water, divided
- 1 cup Cheddar cheese, shredded
- 2 cups rolled oats
- 4 organic eggs, large, cooked
- 2 teaspoons red-wine vinegar
- ¼ cup chipotle salsa, plus more for serving
- 2 tablespoons extra-virgin olive oil, divided
- ½ teaspoon each of ground pepper & salt, divided

Directions:

1. First, over medium heat in a large saucepan; heat 1 tablespoon of oil until hot; swirl to coat the bottom of your pan completely. Add shallot, then cook for a minute or two, until softened, stirring every now and then. Add and stir the oats for a minute. Add 4 of cups water & ¼ teaspoon each of pepper and salt. Bring the mixture to a boil. Once done; decrease the heat & let simmer for 10 to 12 minutes, until creamy, stirring often.

2. Next, in the meantime, over medium-high heat in a large skillet; heat the leftover oil until hot. Add collards with the leftover water and ¼ teaspoon each pepper and salt; give the ingredients a good stir. Then, cook for a couple of more minutes, until turn tender, stirring occasionally. Remove from the heat and then, stir in the vinegar.

3. Stir salsa and cheese into the oatmeal. Serve immediately and enjoy.

Nutritional Value: kcal: 410, Fat: 24 g, Fiber: 8 g, Protein: 21 g, Carbohydrates: 30 g

Cocoa-Chia Pudding with Raspberries

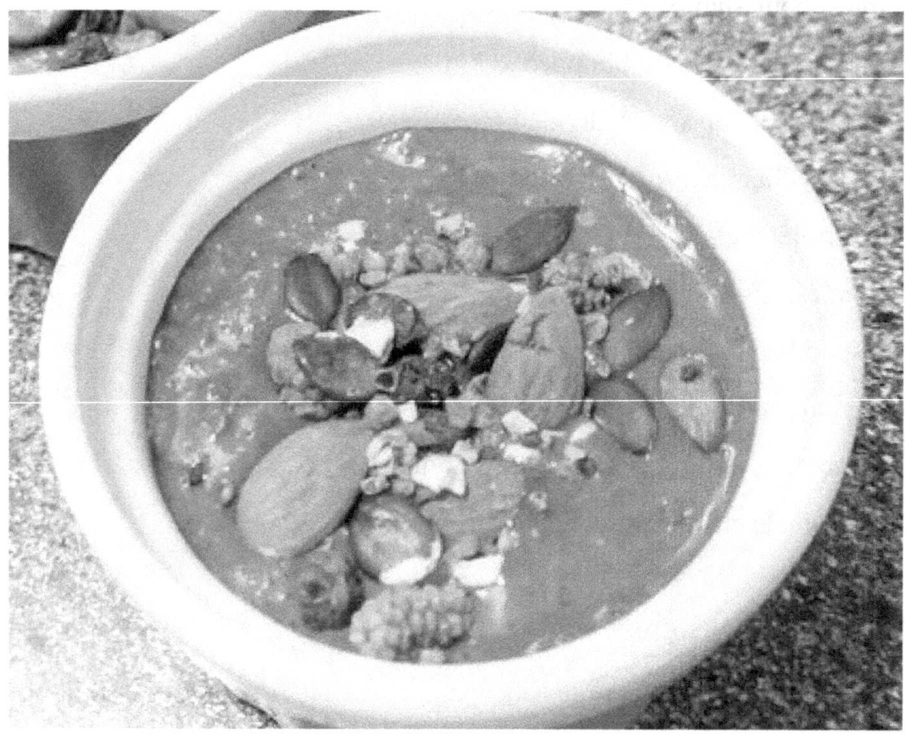

Prep Time: 10 minutes

Cooking Time: 8 hours & 15 minutes

Servings: 1 person

If you are looking for a chocolate treat breakfast recipe, I strongly recommend you prepare this. This is certainly one of my favorite breakfast recipes that I often prepare for my loved ones. For a nice crunch, you can use cacao nibs instead of cocoa powder.

Ingredients:

- ½ cup raspberries, fresh, divided
- ¼ teaspoon vanilla extract
- 2 teaspoons pure maple syrup
- 2 tablespoons chia seeds
- 1 tablespoon toasted sliced almonds, then divided
- ½ cup almond milk, unsweetened
- ½ teaspoon cocoa powder, unsweetened

Directions:

1. First, stir almond milk with maple syrup, chia, vanilla and cocoa in your small-sized mixing bowl. Cover & let refrigerate for overnight.

2. The next morning; give the ingredients a good stir. Spoon approximately half of the prepared pudding into your serving bowl or glass & top with half of the almonds and raspberries. Add the remaining pudding and then, top with the leftover almonds and raspberries.

Nutritional Value: kcal: 220, Fat: 11 g, Fiber: 12 g, Protein: 6 g, Carbohydrates: 27 g

Baby Kale Salad with Quinoa & Strawberries

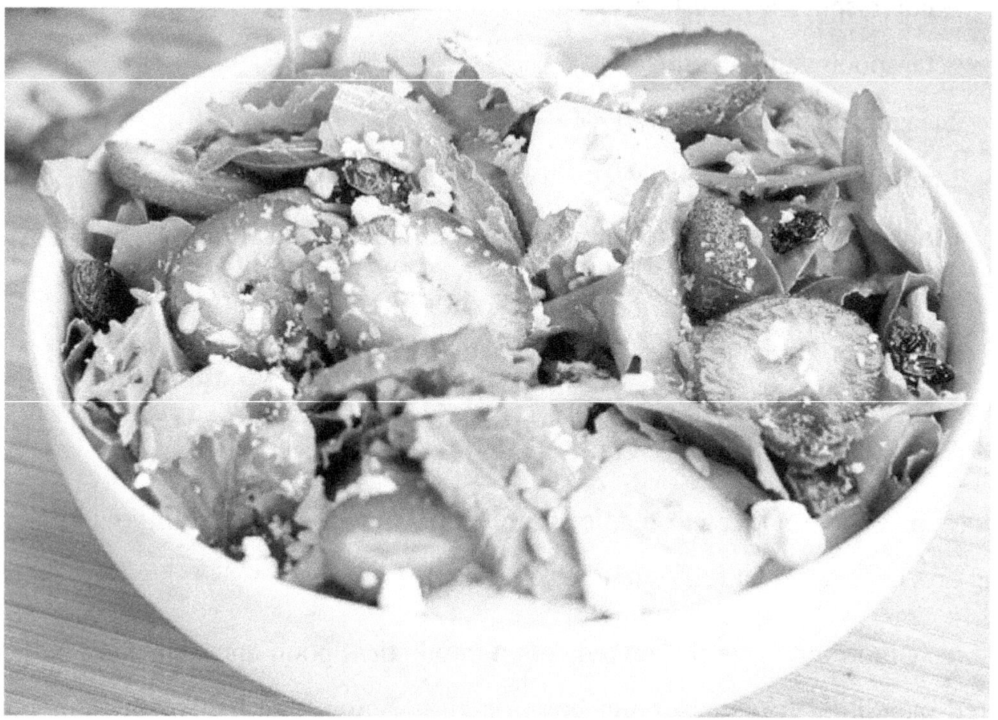

Prep Time: 10 minutes

Cooking Time: 15 minutes

Servings: 1 person

Looking for a salad recipe with green leafy kale, then you must go for this one. This recipe would keep your tummy full for several hours, and you won't need anything else. You can squeeze a fresh lemon and sprinkle some black pepper on top. Enjoy.

Ingredients:

- 1 teaspoon garlic, minced
- 2 teaspoons red-wine vinegar
- ½ cup strawberries, sliced
- 3 cups baby kale, lightly packed
- 1 tablespoon salted pepitas
- ½ cup quinoa, cooked
- 1 tablespoon extra-virgin olive oil
- A pinch each of ground pepper & salt

Directions:

1. Mash the garlic & salt using the side of a fork or a chef's knife until you get paste like consistency. Whisk garlic paste with vinegar, oil & pepper in a medium-sized mixing bowl. Add kale; generously toss to coat. Serve immediately topped with strawberries, quinoa & pepitas.

Nutritional Value: kcal: 300, Fat: 20 g, Fiber: 6 g, Protein: 9 g, Carbohydrates: 31 g

Lunch

Shredded Chicken with Vegetable Broth

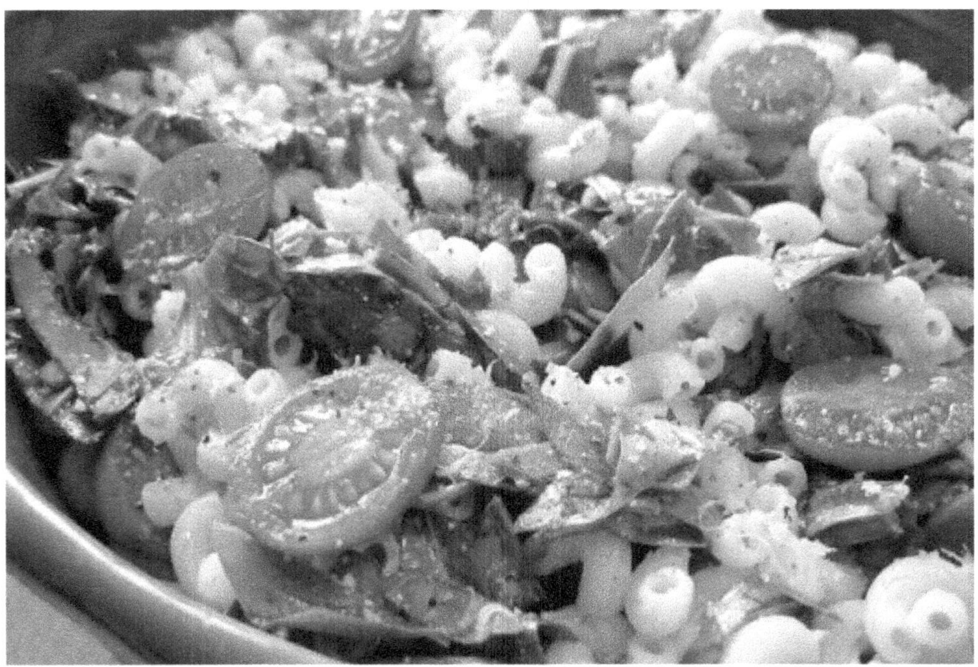

Prep Time: 10 minutes

Cooking Time: 10 minutes

Servings: 2 persons

A nice and delicious recipe that you can try for your lunch. You can substitute the spring greens with ½ savory cabbage and add some cooked broccoli as well. For added crunch, you can even top each bowl with some crunchy Parmesan toasts or finish each bowl with pesto.

Ingredients:

- 1 slice sourdough bread, cut into cubes
- 3 cups chicken stock
- 1 large chicken breast, skin on
- 2 tablespoons parmesan, grated
- ¼ cup peas, fresh or frozen
- 2 large handfuls of spring greens, nicely sliced
- 1 can borlotti beans, drained & rinsed (approximately 1 pound)
- 4 asparagus spears, trimmed, halved & cut into chunky pieces
- 1 tablespoon olive oil

Directions:

1. Preheat your oven to 405 F in advance. Next, over moderate heat in a large pan; heat 1 teaspoon of oil until hot and cook the chicken until turn brown, then remove it from the heat source and transfer the content to a large-sized bowl. Now fill the same pan with the stock and bring it to a boil over moderate heat. Once done, add the chicken & cook for a couple of minutes. Cover with a lid and turn the heat off; let stand for half an hour.

2. Spread the bread cubes on a large-sized baking tray and then, drizzle with the leftover oil, some Parmesan and salt. Bake until crunchy & turn golden, for a couple of more minutes. Remove & scrapping anything leftover on the tray to a large plate.

3. Remove the chicken from pan & slice it. Heat the stock again and bring it to a boil. Once done; add the greens, peas and asparagus. Cook for a minute and add the chicken and beans. Continue to cook until heated through and then, pour into individual bowls; top each bowl with the Parmesan toast; serve immediately & enjoy.

Nutritional Value: kcal: 465, Fat: 17 g, Fiber: 12 g, Protein: 43 g, Carbohydrates: 28 g

Delicious Kale Recipe

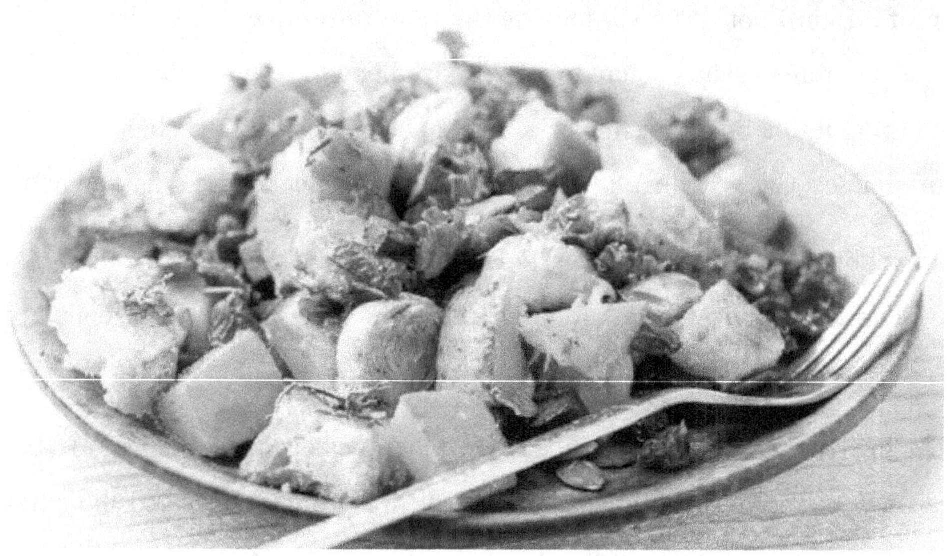

Prep Time: 10 minutes

Cooking Time: 20 minutes

Servings: 2 persons

This recipe is simply delicious and quite easy to prepare. You can customize it per your preference. You can even use 1 teaspoon of ground cumin than the seeds, a sachet of creamed coconut and skip the ginger.

Ingredients:

- 1 onion, finely chopped
- 2 heaped teaspoons cumin seeds
- 1 teaspoon turmeric
- 2 tablespoons tomato purée
- 1 ½ cups kale, remove the large stalks, finely shred the leaves
- thumb-sized piece ginger, grated
- 1 can chickpeas, drained (approximately 1 pound)
- 2 cups vegetable stock
- 1 teaspoon ground coriander
- 50g fresh coconut, grated or desiccated coconut
- 1 tablespoon butter
- 4 heaped tablespoons Greek-style yogurt
- 1 tablespoon fresh mango chutney

To serve

- 2 tablespoons freeze-dried curry leaves
- 1 tablespoon vegetable oil
- 3 garlic cloves, sliced thinly

Directions:

1. Over moderate heat in a deep-frying pan; heat the butter until melted, then add the onion. Cook for 3 to 5 minutes, until turn soften. Increase the heat; add the ginger followed by the spices; continue to fry the ingredients until garlic turns fragrant, for a minute or two more and then, stir in the tomato purée.

2. Next, add the kale followed by chickpeas, two-thirds of the coconut and stock; give the ingredients a good stir and then, cover the pan with a lid. Bring the mixture to a simmer. Once done; decrease the heat and let steam until wilted, for 8 to 10 minutes. Mix in the chutney and yogurt, then season to taste (ensure that you don't bring the mixture to a boil this time). Remove the pan from heat & set aside (covered).

3. Now, over moderate heat in a small saucepan; heat the oil until hot. When done, add the garlic followed by the curry leaves; cook until the garlic starts to turn golden, for a minute. Spoon the garlic, curry leaves & oil on top of the kale and chickpeas, then finish the cooking process with the leftover coconut.

Nutritional Value: kcal: 220, Fat: 10 g, Fiber: 6 g, Protein: 10 g, Carbohydrates: 21 g

Stir-Fried Broccoli with Coconut

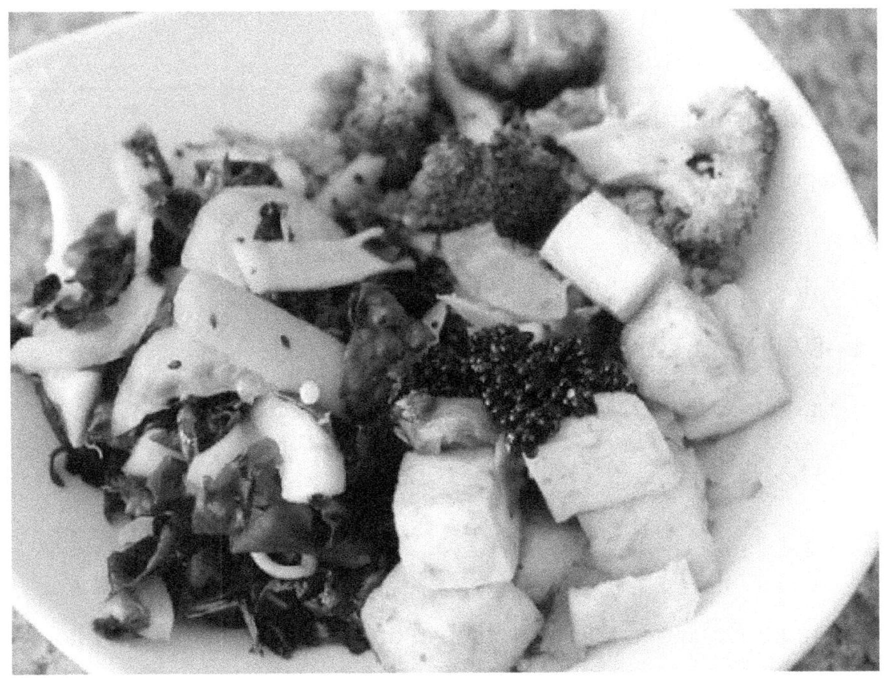

Prep Time: 10 minutes

Cooking Time: 10 minutes

Servings: 10 persons

A healthy way to get some greens into your diet! You can prepare this recipe with some cabbage or sprouts. You can even use some frozen grated coconut as well. If you are using desiccated coconut (3 tablespoons), then you need to soak it in hot water for a couple of minutes approximately before using it.

Ingredients:

- 2 pounds thin-stemmed broccoli, cut into bite-sized pieces
- 3½ teaspoons mustard seed
- 4oz grated coconut, fresh or frozen
- 3 tablespoons curry leaf, fresh or dried
- 100g ginger, shredded
- 4 red onions, sliced thickly
- Juice of 2 limes, freshly squeezed
- 6 tablespoons vegetable oil
- A pinch of chili flakes

Directions:

1. First, over a medium heat in a large saucepan or wok; heat the oil until hot. Once done; toss the mustard seeds and then add the curry leaves and chili flakes; give the ingredients a good swirl until the leaves stop spluttering. Next, add onions & ginger; continue to stir-fry over a high heat for 3 to 4 minutes.

2. Stir in the broccoli & the dried curry leaves; continue to fry until just tender, stirring frequently. Scatter over the coconut; give the ingredients a good stir until mixed well and squeeze the lime juice on top. Serve hot & enjoy.

Nutritional Value: kcal: 150, Fat: 12 g, Fiber: 4 g, Protein: 5 g, Carbohydrates: 7 g

Chicken with Added Vegetables and Nuts

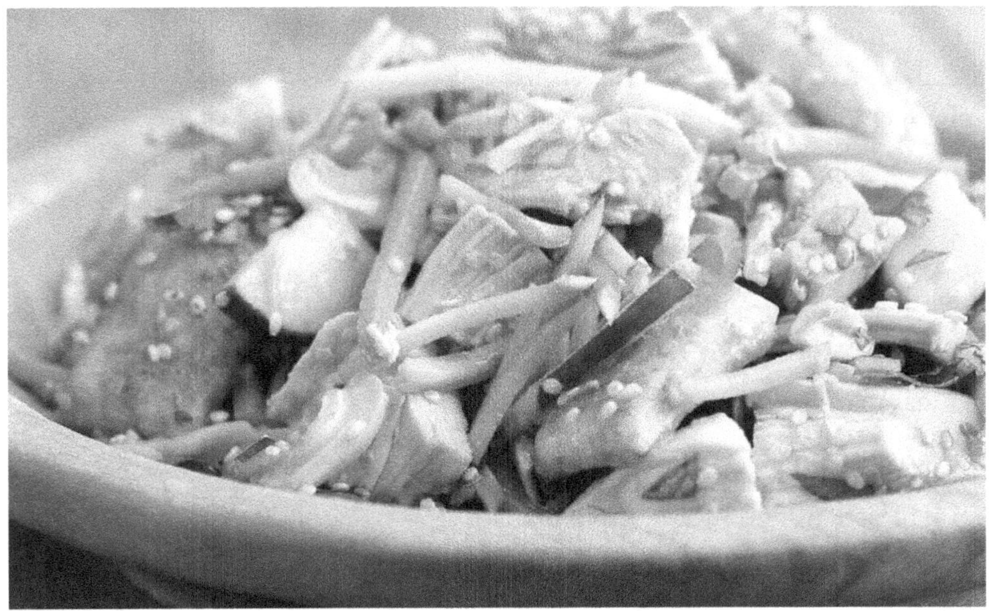

Prep Time: 10 minutes

Cooking Time: 25 minutes

Servings: 2 persons

This recipe is a super healthy meal and has plenty of Vitamin C. You can skip the lemon zest and add some soy and chili to it. Just add a bit of fresh ginger and serve it with some egg noodles.

Ingredients:

- 1 pack tender stem broccoli (approximately ½ pound), stems halved
- 2 cloves garlic, sliced
- 1 ½ cups chicken stock
- 1 pack mini chicken breast fillets (approximately 1 pound)
- Zest of ½ lemon, fresh
- 1 heaped teaspoon corn flour
- Juice of 1 lemon, fresh
- 2 teaspoons golden caster sugar or 1 tablespoon clear honey
- 1 large handful of cashews, roasted
- 1 tablespoon sunflower or groundnut oil

Directions:

1. First, over moderate heat in a wok or large frying pan; heat the oil until hot. Add and fry the chicken until turn golden, for 3 to 4 minutes. Remove the chicken pieces & add broccoli and garlic to the hot pan. Stir fry the ingredients for a minute; cover & continue to cook until almost tender, for 2 more minutes.

2. Next, add the stock followed by sugar or honey and corn flour in a large bowl; mix well and then, pour the mixture into the hot pan & stir the ingredients until thickened, for a couple of minutes. Tip the chicken into the hot pan again & continue to cook until heated through. Add the lemon juice and zest followed by the cashew nuts. Give the ingredients a good stir; serve immediately with some noodles or basmati rice and enjoy.

Nutritional Value: kcal: 370, Fat: 13 g, Fiber: 3 g, Protein: 48 g, Carbohydrates: 15 g

Spinach & Watercress Salad

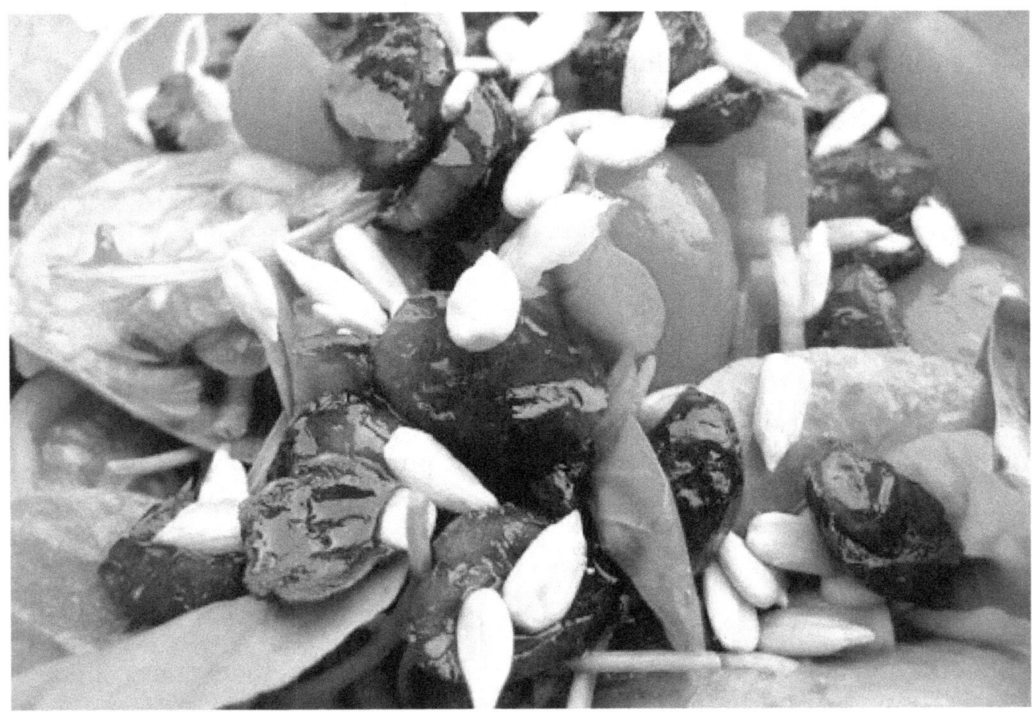

Prep Time: 10 minutes

Cooking Time: 10 minutes

Servings: 4 persons

This recipe is absolutely healthy, and you would get plenty of Vitamin C from it. If desired, you can even add a bit of balsamic vinegar to enhance the taste.

Ingredients:

- 100g bag baby spinach leaves, washed & cleaned
- 1 small red onion, finely sliced
- Lemon juice, freshly squeezed, to taste
- 2 tablespoons extra-virgin olive oil
- 1 large bunch of watercress, stalks trimmed

Directions:

1. Whisk lemon juice with oil and then, season to taste. Combine the leaves with onion in a large-sized mixing bowl and then, drizzle the prepared dressing on top; toss until combined well. Serve immediately & enjoy.

Nutritional Value: kcal: 66, Fat: 6 g, Fiber: 1 g, Protein: 3 g, Carbohydrates: 2 g

Zesty Salmon with Roasted Beets & Spinach

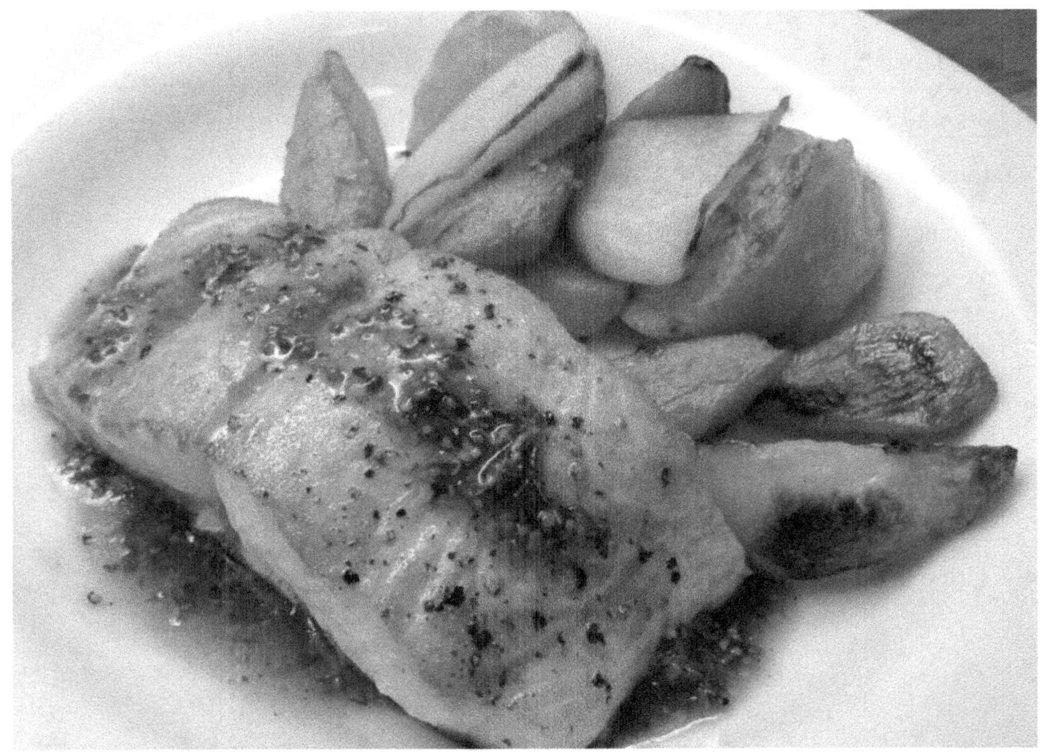

Prep Time: 10 minutes

Cooking Time: 50 minutes

Servings: 2 persons

This recipe is a great source of calcium, vitamin C and iron. It tastes great and easy to prepare. You can sub the pumpkin seeds with roasted almonds.

Ingredients:

- 2 skinless salmon or trout fillets
- 1½ tablespoons rapeseed oil
- 4 small fresh beetroots, approximately ½ pound; stems trimmed & reserving the tender leaves
- 1 teaspoon coriander seeds, lightly crushed
- 2½ small oranges, zest of 1 & juice of remaining
- 1 red onion, finely chopped
- 1 garlic clove
- 3 tablespoons pumpkin seeds
- 4 handfuls of fresh baby spinach leaves
- 1 ripe avocado, thickly sliced

Directions:

1. Preheat your oven to 360 F in advance.

2. Cut the beetroots into quarters and then toss with ½ tablespoon of oil followed by some seasoning, and coriander seeds, then pile into the middle of a large-sized aluminum foil sheet; wrap up just like you would with a parcel. Bake in your preheated oven until tender, for 40 to 45 minutes. Top with the salmon fillets; scatter half of the orange zest on top and bake for 12 to 15 more minutes. If desired, feel free to toast the pumpkin seeds for 8 to 10 minutes.

3. In the meantime; cut the peel & pith from 2 oranges; cut the segments out using a sharp knife (catch up the juices in a large bowl). Finely grate the garlic; set aside for 8 to 10 minutes. Next, prepare the dressing by stirring the garlic in the freshly squeezed orange juice and leftover oil with the seasoning.

4. Remove the parcel from oven & carefully remove the fish; tipping the beetroot into a bowl with the remaining orange zest, red onion, spinach leaves and pumpkin seeds; toss well.

5. Gently toss through the avocado and orange segments along with any beet leaves and then, pile on the plates; topping the recipe with the hot salmon. Drizzle with dressing; serve immediately and enjoy.

Nutritional Value: kcal: 543, Fat: 32 g, Fiber: 10 g, Protein: 35 g, Carbohydrates: 25 g

Trout with Almonds & Red Peppers

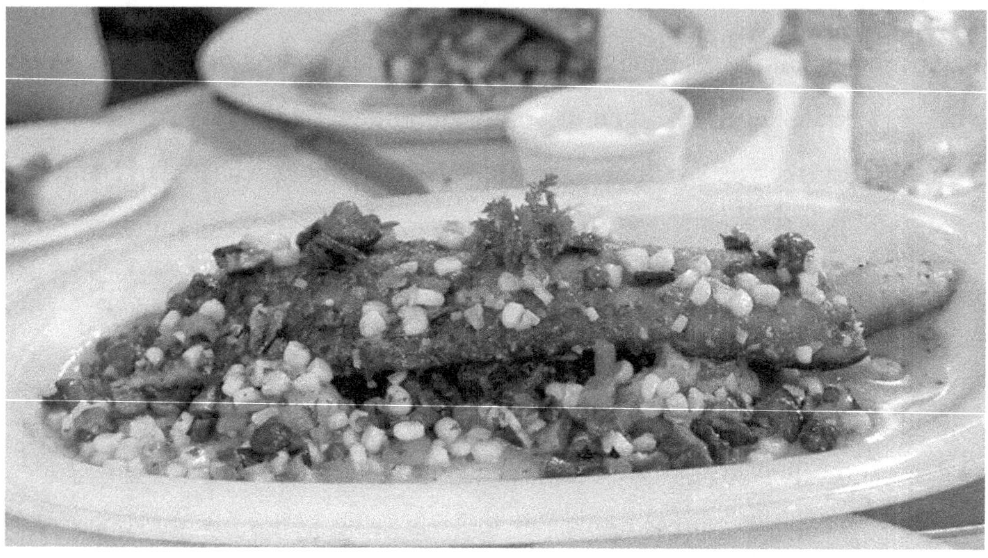

Prep Time: 10 minutes

Cooking Time: 35 minutes

Servings: 2 persons

This recipe is flavorful and quite delicious too. You can try trout instead of salmon. You can add fennel to the roast and serve with new potatoes and asparagus.

Ingredients:

- 1 garlic clove, chopped
- 2 trout fillets, approximately 140g each
- 1 tablespoon balsamic vinegar
- 1 handful of cherry tomatoes, halved or 2 large tomatoes, roughly chopped
- 1 large red pepper, deseeded & chopped
- 2 tablespoons flaked almonds
- 1 tablespoon olive oil, plus a little

To Serve

- Lemon wedges & rocket salad

Directions:

1. Preheat your oven to 380 F in advance.

2. Tip the tomatoes with pepper, garlic, vinegar and oil into a roasting tin and then toss well until nicely mixed. Roast for 17 to 20 minutes in the preheated oven.

3. Once done; make some space in the roasting tin and then add the trout fillets, spreading some almonds on top and a small amount of pepper and salt.

4. Bake in the oven again until the almonds are toasted lightly and the fish is completely cooked through, for 12 to 15 minutes more. Serve with a rocket salad and lemon wedges on the side. Enjoy.

Nutritional Value: kcal: 320, Fat: 17 g, Fiber: 3 g, Protein: 31 g, Carbohydrates: 11 g

Gingery Shiitake Noodles

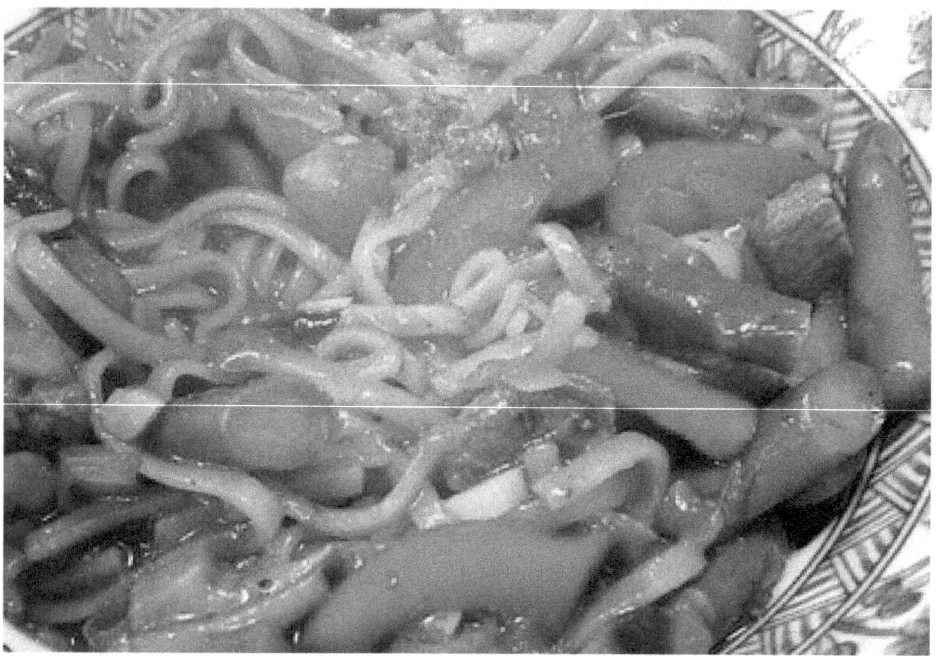

Prep Time: 10 minutes

Cooking Time: 15 minutes

Servings: 8 persons

If you love noodles and are looking for a noodle recipe, then you should go for this one. You would fall in love with this recipe. You can even use dried Shitake mushrooms, and the taste would still remain the same. For more heat, just add some slices of fresh chili. Serve and enjoy.

Ingredients:

- 1 pack medium dried egg noodle (approximately 1 pound)
- 2 tablespoons light soy sauce
- A few dashes of sesame oil, toasted
- 8 spring onions, cut into 1/3, then sliced thinly into strips lengthways
- Fresh root ginger, grated, preferably finger-length piece
- 2 tablespoons oyster sauce
- ¾ pound shiitake mushroom, fresh, sliced
- 2 tablespoons groundnut oil

Directions:

1. Prepare the noodles per the instructions mentioned on the package and then toss with a small amount of sesame oil (ensure that they don't stick together).

2. Now, over high heat in a wok; heat the groundnut oil until hot & smoky. Once done, add & stir-fry the ginger for a few seconds and then, add the mushrooms with a splash of water; cook for a minute. Toss the cooked noodles until hot, for a couple of minutes and then, add the soy and oyster sauces, spring onions & a dash of more sesame oil. Serve immediately & enjoy.

Nutritional Value: kcal: 225, Fat: 8 g, Fiber: 2 g, Protein: 7 g, Carbohydrates: 35 g

Roast Brill with Puy Lentils & Shiitake Mushrooms

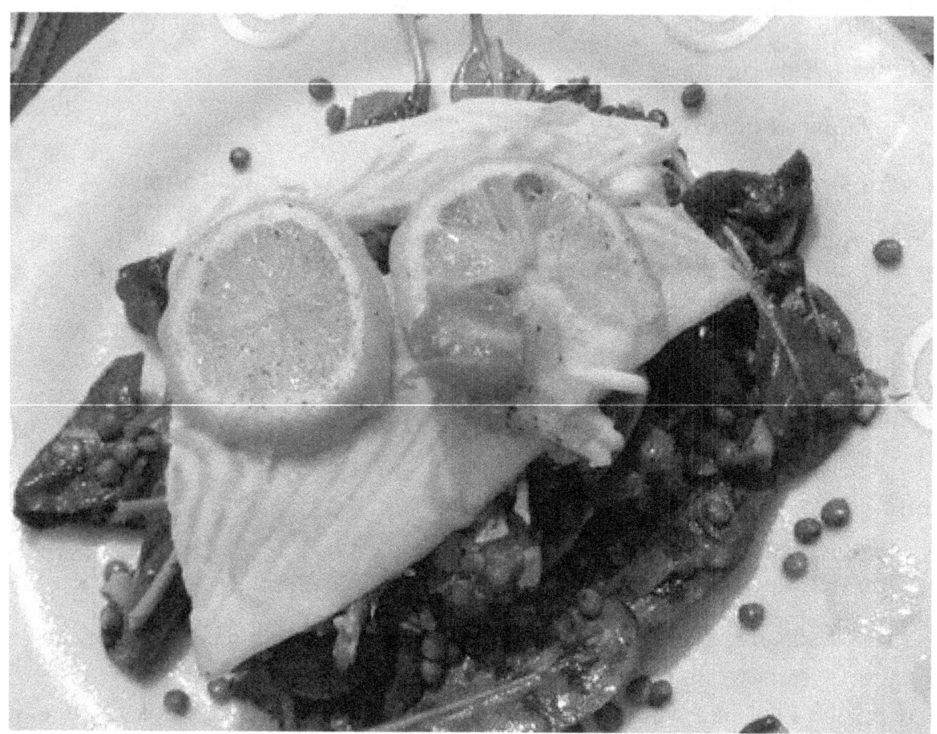

Prep Time: 10 minutes

Cooking Time: 40 minutes

Servings: 4 persons

This recipe tastes great and quite easy to prepare. My family loved it and asked me to serve the remaining in the dinner. Just before serving, I squeezed a fresh lemon on top and it was a hit.

Ingredients:

- 4 x brill fillets, skinned (approximately 140g each)
- ¼ pound shiitake mushroom, quartered
- 2 shallots, finely chopped
- 1 cup white wine
- ½ pound plum or cherry tomatoes, halved
- 1 bunch of flat-leaf parsley, roughly chopped
- 2 tablespoons capers, rinsed
- 4 tablespoons olive oil
- 1 cup baby spinach leaves, fresh
- ½ pound pun lentils
- 1 small lemon, thinly sliced

Directions:

1. Preheat your oven to 405 F in advance.

2. Cover a large pan with water and add the lentils (ensure that they are completely covered). Then, bring it to a boil over moderate heat & continue to cook until tender, for 15 to 20 minutes. Drain well & set aside.

3. Now, over moderate heat in a large pan; heat half of the oil and fry the shallots until softened, for a couple of minutes. Increase the heat & add the mushrooms; continue to cook until the edges turn browned, for a couple of minutes. Then, remove it from the heat. Stir in the halved tomatoes, cooked lentils, capers & wine; give the ingredients a good stir until nicely mixed.

4. Place the fish fillets over the hot lentils and then top with a few slices of lemon; drizzle with the leftover oil and then, season with the freshly ground black pepper and flaked sea salt. Then, roast until the fish is cooked through and beginning to go golden on top, for 12 to 15 minutes.

5. Gently lift the fish from pan & stir the spinach and parsley into the lentils; cook for a couple of more minutes approximately, until the spinach begins to wilt. Evenly spoon the mixture among 4 plates; place the fish fillet on top; serve immediately & enjoy.

Nutritional Value: kcal: 470, Fat: 17 g, Fiber: 5 g, Protein: 42 g, Carbohydrates: 30 g

Sea Bass with Sizzled Ginger, Chili & Spring Onions

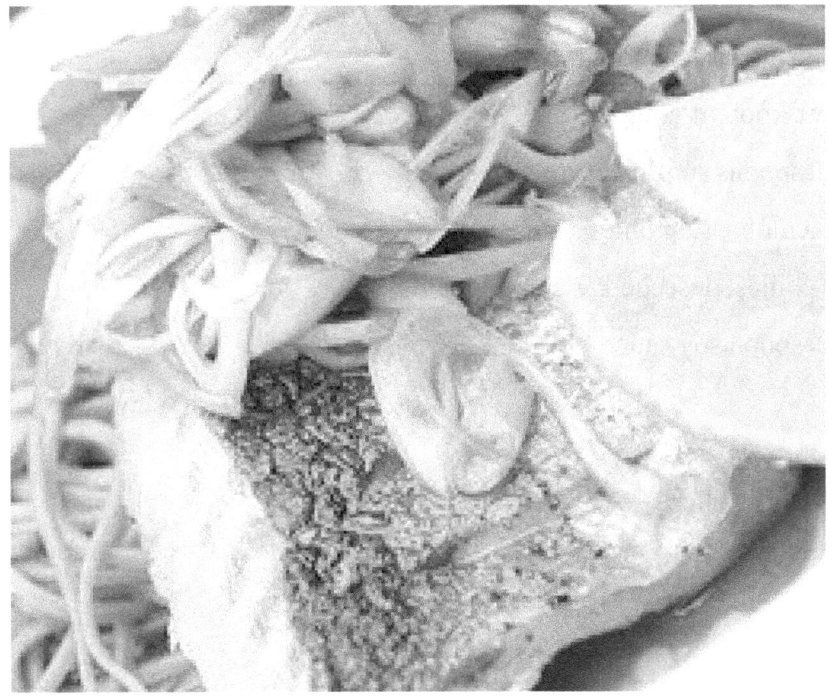

Prep Time: 15 minutes

Cooking Time: 15 minutes

Servings: 6 persons

This recipe has a lot of flavors and it's quite easy to prepare as well. Just serve it with fried potatoes & broccoli or broccoli stems, Asparagus & boiled rice. Enjoy the taste.

Ingredients:

- 6 sea bass fillets, skin on & scaled (approximately 5oz each)
- 3 garlic cloves, sliced thinly
- A large knob of ginger, peeled & shredded into matchsticks
- 3 tablespoons sunflower oil
- A bunch of spring onion, shredded
- 3 red chilies; deseeded & shredded thinly
- 1 tablespoon soy sauce

Directions:

1. Season the sea bass fillets with pepper and salt then slice the skin a couple of times.

2. Now, over moderate heat in a heavy-based frying pan; heat 1 tablespoon of sunflower oil until hot.

3. Once done, work in batches and fry the sea bass fillets until the skin turns golden and is very crisp, for 3 to 5 minutes, skin-side down.

4. Carefully turn the fish over & continue to cook for 30 seconds to 1 minute more; transfer to a large-sized serving plate & keep it warm.

5. Now, heat 2 tablespoons of sunflower oil and fry the matchsticks of ginger followed by garlic cloves (thinly sliced) & red chilies (thinly shredded) until turn golden, for 2 more minutes.

6. Remove from the heat & toss in the bunch of shredded spring onions. Add approximately 1 tablespoon of the soy sauce on top of the fish & spoon over the ingredients inside the pan.

Nutritional Value: kcal: 200, Fat: 8 g, Fiber: 1 g, Protein: 28 g, Carbohydrates: 2 g

Dinner

Chicken with Brazil Nuts & Pomegranate

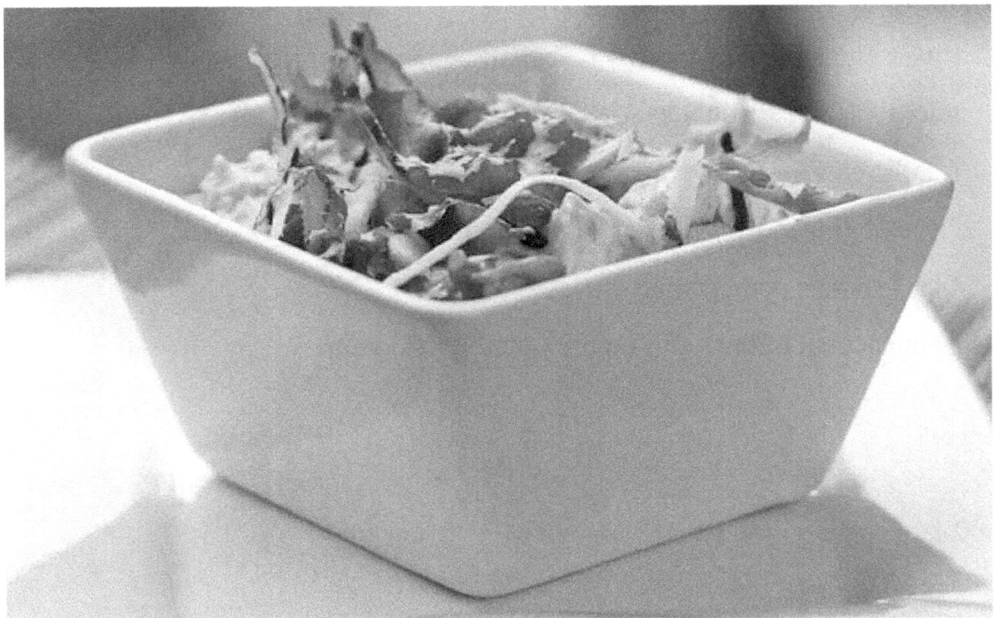

Prep Time: 35 minutes

Cooking Time: 50 minutes

Servings: 6 persons

For a mouth-watering dinner, just marinate the chicken in ginger, pomegranate molasses and lime, serve on a few slices of aubergine (preferably grilled) or serve with rice salad and grated courgette.

Ingredients:

- 6 chicken quarters or legs, free-range
- 1 pack Brazil nuts, half left whole, half chopped (approximately 150 grams)
- Juice of 1 lime, freshly squeezed
- 1 garlic clove
- Piece of ginger, peeled (preferably thumb-sized)
- 4 tablespoons pomegranate molasses
- 1 pot coconut milk yogurt (approximately 250grams)

To Serve:

- 2 large aubergines, lengthways sliced
- 1 pomegranate, only seeds
- 2 tablespoons rapeseed oil

Directions:

1. Blend the ginger with whole Brazil nuts, lime juice and garlic in a food processor until you get paste like consistency then add the molasses and coconut yogurt. Blend again and then add the mixture along with the chicken into a large-sized mixing bowl. Mix well until nicely coated in the marinade. Using a cling film; cover the bowl & leave in the fridge for overnight.

2. The next day, preheat your oven to 380 F in advance. Spread the chicken, skin-side up in a deep roasting tin & cook in the preheated oven until turn golden brown & juices run clear, for 45 to 55 minutes

3. In the meantime, coat the aubergine slices lightly with oil & cook until tender and patterned with char marks, for 3 to 4 minutes per side, on a hot griddle pan. Arrange the aubergines on a large-sized serving platter; add the cooked chicken & scatter the pomegranate seeds and chopped Brazil nuts on top.

Nutritional Value: kcal: 700, Fat: 40 g, Fiber: 2 g, Protein: 45 g, Carbohydrates: 4 g

Delicious Salad with Tangy Dressing

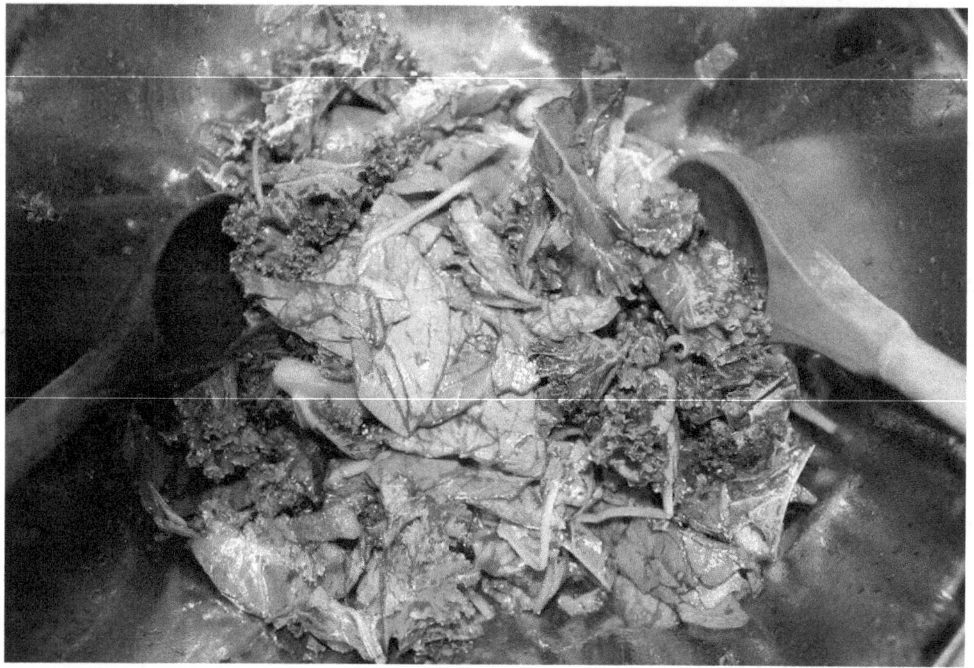

Prep Time: 20 minutes

Cooking Time: 10 minutes

Servings: 6 persons

If you want something warm, hearty, and crunchy salad, then you can always go for this recipe. This salad recipe is doable and packed with healthy nutrients. Serve, garnished with fresh cilantro, and enjoy.

Ingredients:

- 1 cup baby spinach, fresh
- ½ pound purple sprouting broccoli, cut into bite-sized chunks or in half
- 1 pouch quinoa, cooked (250g)
- 175g soya bean, frozen
- 1 cup pomegranate seeds
- 2 ripe avocados
- 1 cup pumpkin seed, toasted in a dry pan until popped
- A handful of soft herbs such as basil, parsley, mint or coriander, chopped

For Citrus Dressing:

- Juice & zest of 1 lime or lemon, freshly squeezed
- 2 tablespoons Dijon mustard
- 1 tablespoon white wine vinegar
- 2 tablespoons extra-virgin rapeseed oil
- Juice & zest of 1 orange, freshly squeezed

Directions:

1. First, fill your large saucepan with cold water and bring it to a boil over moderate heat. Once boiling; add the broccoli & cook for a couple of minutes and then, add the soya beans; continue to cook until the broccoli is almost cooked, for 1 to 2 more minutes. Drain & drop the vegetables into the cold water. Leave until cool, for a couple of minutes and then, drain; leave in the colander.

2. Add the seasoning with dressing ingredients in a large bowl; mix well using a whisk. Halve, stone & peel the avocados; cutting them into chunky dice & add into the dressing mixture. Add the spinach, quinoa, half the pomegranate, pumpkin seeds, herbs and the cooked vegetables to the bowl; toss gently. Transfer the prepared salad to a serving platter; scatter with the leftover seeds; serve immediately & enjoy.

Nutritional Value: kcal: 330, Fat: 25 g, Fiber: 5 g, Protein: 16 g, Carbohydrates: 20 g

Roasted Cauliflower Tabbouleh

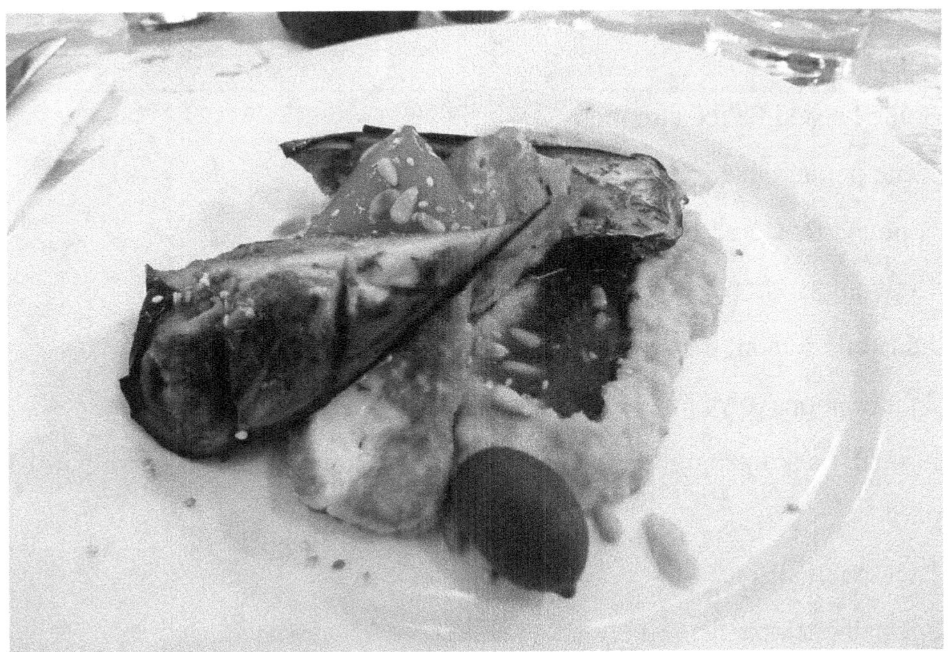

Prep Time: 10 minutes

Cooking Time: 20 minutes

Servings: 4 persons

You can prepare this grain-free, low-calorie meal with roasted cauliflower, sweet pomegranate seeds and punchy feta in advance. If you don't want to use allspice, then just mix some spices & add black pepper. You can finely chop the spring onions and replace the almonds with some toasted pine nuts.

Ingredients:

- 1 large cauliflower (approximately 1 ½ pounds); outer leaves & hard inner core removed
- Some toasted flaked almonds
- 1 cup pomegranate seeds
- ½ pound feta, crumbled, packed
- 1 red onion, chopped finely
- Juice of 1 lemon, freshly squeezed
- 2 tablespoons olive oil
- ½ small pack fresh mint, chopped finely, plus some fresh leaves for garnish purpose
- 1 teaspoon allspice
- ½ small pack parsley, finely chopped
- 1 teaspoon ground cinnamon

Directions:

1. Preheat your oven to 405 F in advance.

2. Chop the florets roughly and then, add them into the food processor; pulse on high power until you get couscous grains like consistency, for 30 seconds and then, tip the mixture to a large-sized mixing bowl.

3. Combine the olive oil and spices to the cauliflower then, season with pepper & salt to taste. Evenly spread the couscous over a baking tray, preferably large-sized. Then, roast in your preheated oven for 10 to 12 minutes, mixing halfway; once done, set aside & let slightly cool.

4. Once done, stir the leftover ingredients & season with pepper & salt to taste. Just before serving; sprinkle some fresh mint leaves on top.

Nutritional Value: kcal: 310, Fat: 15 g, Fiber: 5 g, Protein: 16 g, Carbohydrates: 14 g

Coconut & Squash Dhansak

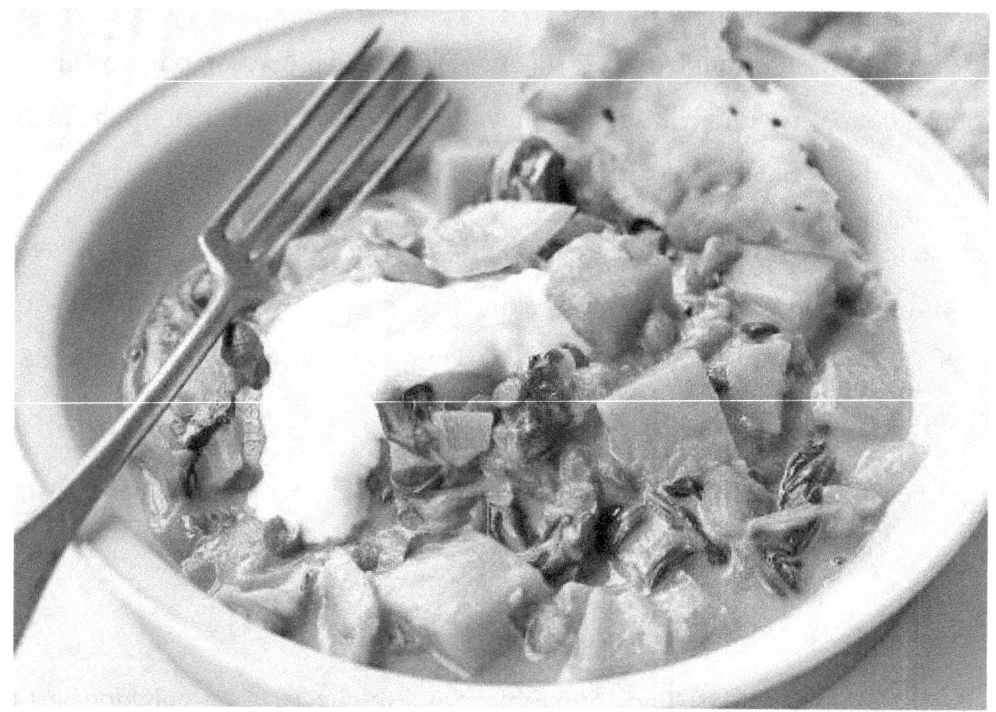

Prep Time: 10 minutes

Cooking Time: 20 minutes

Servings: 4 persons

This recipe tastes great and quite easy to prepare. While preparing, I added a few red pepper and spring onions. Serve this recipe with some Indian Naan or freshly prepared green mint chutney.

Ingredients:

- 1 ¼ pounds butternut squash, peeled & chopped into bite-sized chunks
- 1 can chopped tomatoes (approximately 1 pound)
- 4 heaping tablespoons mild curry paste
- 1 cup coconut yogurt, plus extra to serve
- 1 can lentils, drained (approximately 1 pound)
- 1 cup onions, chopped, frozen
- ½ pound bag baby spinach, fresh
- 1 can light coconut milk (approximately 1 pound)
- 1 tablespoon vegetable oil

Directions:

1. Over moderate heat in a large pan; heat the oil until hot. Add squash with a splash of water in a large-sized mixing bowl. Using a cling film; cover & microwave until tender, for 8 to 10 minutes, on High power. In the meantime, carefully add onions into the hot oil & cook until soft, for a couple of minutes. Add the tomatoes, curry paste and coconut milk, let simmer until thickened, for 8 to 10 minutes.

2. Next, warm the naan breads in the toaster or in a lower rack of your oven. Drain any liquid from the squash; add it to the sauce with the spinach, lentils and some of the seasoning. Let simmer until the spinach wilts, for 2 to 3 more minutes and then stir in the coconut yogurt.

3. Lastly, serve with a dollop of extra yogurt and the warm naan. Enjoy.

Nutritional Value: kcal: 320, Fat: 15 g, Fiber: 7 g, Protein: 10 g, Carbohydrates: 25 g

Grilled Lamb with Wintry Rice Salad

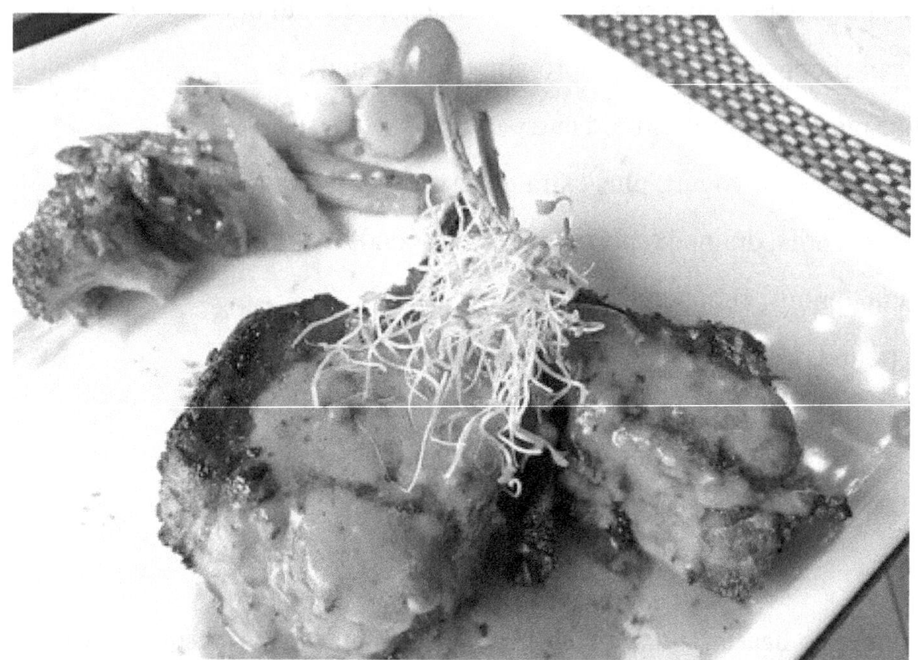

Prep Time: 20 minutes

Cooking Time: 30 minutes

Servings: 4 persons

If you are looking for a healthy dinner recipe, then you must go for this one. This delicious recipe is packed with a sufficient amount of protein and nutrients.

Ingredients:

- 1 pound lean lamb steak
- 2 red onions
- 1 teaspoon cinnamon
- A handful of fresh mint, chopped
- 1 cup pomegranate seeds, fresh
- A handful of fresh parsley, chopped
- 1 cup wild & basmati rice
- 50g cranberries, dried
- Juice of ½ orange, fresh
- 1 tablespoon olive oil
- Juice of ½ lemon, fresh
- 50g pistachio, chopped

Directions:

1. Grate one onion into a shallow dish and then, add ½ tablespoon of olive oil and cinnamon; mix well. Add lamb steaks into the dish; rubbing into the marinade. Cover & set aside while you prepare the rice.

2. Fill a large pan with approximately 600 ml of water and then add the rice. Then, bring it to a boil over moderate heat and decrease the heat; let simmer for 15 - 20 minutes, until the rice absorbs the water, covered. Remove the lid & let cool. In the meantime, finely chop the leftover red onion & mix into the rice with the pomegranate, herbs, cranberries and pistachios. Finally mix in the lemon and orange juice, the leftover olive oil & season to taste.

3. Remove the lamb from marinade, removing any excess marinade. Griddle for 3 to 5 minutes per side. Serve hot with a large spoonful of hot rice.

Nutritional Value: kcal: 490, Fat: 19 g, Fiber: 3 g, Protein: 36 g, Carbohydrates: 35 g

Spiced lamb Kebabs with Pea & Herb Couscous

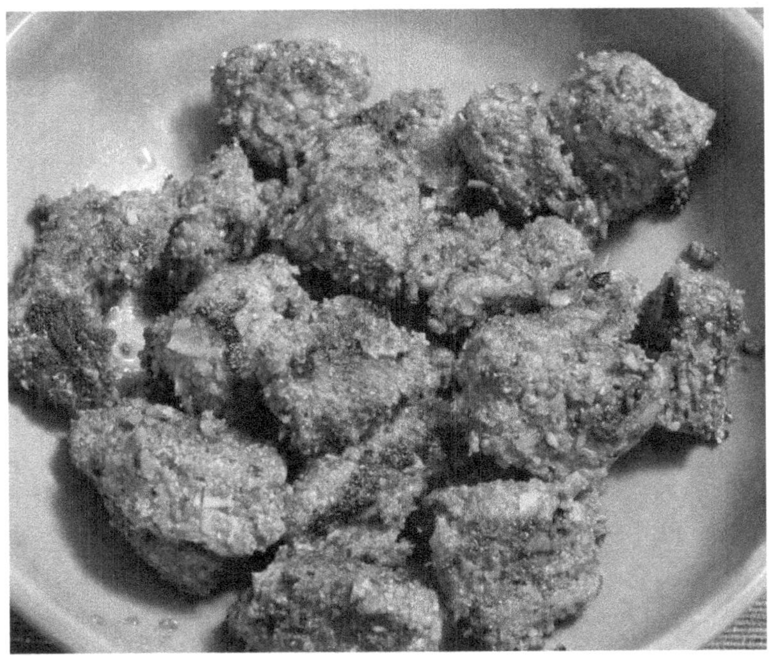

Prep Time: 20 minutes

Cooking Time: 20 minutes

Servings: 3 persons

Absolutely delicious and tempting! I have personally prepared this recipe a lot of times, and each time, it was a hit. I served it with a vegetable couscous flavored with fresh coriander and mint.

Ingredients:

- 1 pound lean lamb shoulder, cut into 3cm cubes
- ½ teaspoon cayenne pepper
- 1 large carrot, coarsely grated
- 24 cherry tomatoes
- 1 teaspoon ground cumin
- 140 g couscous
- 1 teaspoon sweet smoked paprika
- 3 cups hot vegetable stock
- Juice of 1 lemon, freshly squeezed
- 1 cup pea, frozen
- A small pack coriander, chopped
- 1 tablespoon olive oil
- 2 tablespoons extra virgin olive oil
- A small pack of fresh mint, chopped

Directions:

1. First, soak six wooden skewers in hot water for half an hour. Put the lamb cubes with olive oil and the spices in a large bowl. Toss well & then season to taste.

2. Thread a lamb piece onto the skewer and then thread a cherry tomato. Repeat this step until you have 4 cherry tomatoes and 4 lamb pieces to each skewer.

3. In the meantime, add couscous in a large-sized mixing bowl; add the peas & then the hot vegetable stock. Give the ingredients a good stir until nicely mixed. Using a cling film; cover & let soak for a couple of minutes.

4. Heat a griddle pan in advance. When the couscous absorb the liquid, gently fluff up the grains using a large fork & stir in the carrot, olive oil, lemon juice & herbs. Mix everything together and then, season to taste; set aside.

5. Place the prepared skewers over the hot griddle pan & cook for 5 to 6 minutes; carefully turn & cook the other side until the tomatoes and meat are charred &cooked through, for 5 to 6 more minutes. Serve the hot skewers with couscous and enjoy.

Nutritional Value: kcal: 460, Fat: 23 g, Fiber: 7 g, Protein: 28 g, Carbohydrates: 30 g

Hake with stewed peppers

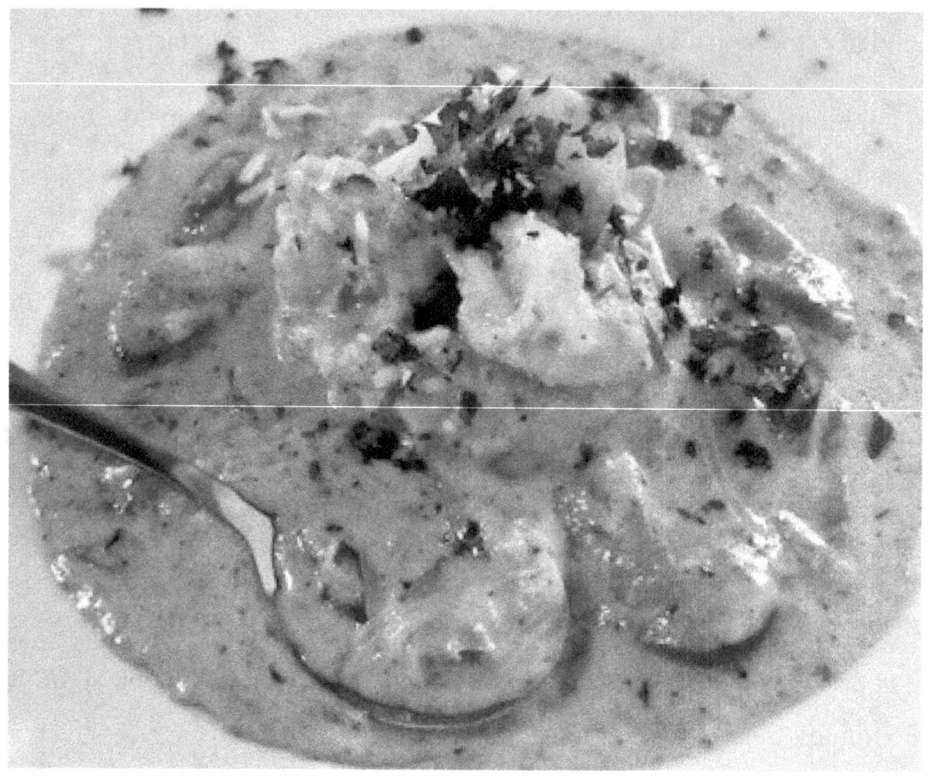

Prep Time: 20 minutes

Cooking Time: 35 minutes

Servings: 4 persons

This is a Spanish-inspired dish and tastes awesome. You would fall in love with the taste and would surely prepare it again for your loved ones on a special day.

Ingredients:

- 4 small cod or hake fillets

- 1 onion, sliced finely

- 3 tablespoons sherry vinegar

- 4 sprigs fresh thyme, remove the leaves but reserve the stems

- 3 peppers, preferably red and yellow each

- 1 tablespoon clear honey

- 2 cloves garlic, chopped

- A small handful of green olives, stoned & halved

- 6 tablespoons extra-virgin olive oil

- 3 tablespoons all-purpose flour

- A large pinch of smoked paprika

Directions:

1. Cook the peppers for a minute or two, until blackened over moderate heat and then put them in a large bowl. Using a cling film; cover & set aside at room temperature until easy to handle. Peel & remove seeds from the peppers and then, strain them into a bowl, preferably small-sized (catching up any juices); set aside and then, cut the flesh into very thin strips & set aside too.

2. Next, over low heat in a shallow pan; heat 3 tablespoons of olive oil until hot. Once done; carefully add onion with thyme stems & garlic; cook until softened & beginning to turn brown, for 15 to 20 minutes. Add the thin pepper strips followed by half of the pepper juice, half of the honey & 2 tablespoons of the Sherry vinegar; cook until you get sticky relish like consistency. Season with paprika; give the ingredients a good stir; adding the olives & set aside.

3. For dressing: Combine the leftover pepper juices with honey, vinegar, 2 tablespoons of olive oil & half of the thyme leaves; mix well & set aside.

4. Toss the all-purpose flour with remaining thyme leaves; add some seasoning. Now, over moderate heat in a non-stick, large frying pan; heat the leftover olive oil & carefully fry the cod or hake, skin-side down for 6 to 8 minutes, until turn golden; carefully flip & continue frying for a couple of more minutes, until completely cooked through. Spoon some of the prepared pepper mix over each plate & top with a piece of cooked cod or hake and then, drizzle the plate with the dressing; serve immediately & enjoy.

Nutritional Value: kcal: 390, Fat: 21 g, Fiber: 5 g, Protein: 23 g, Carbohydrates: 20 g

Speedy Lamb & Spinach Curry

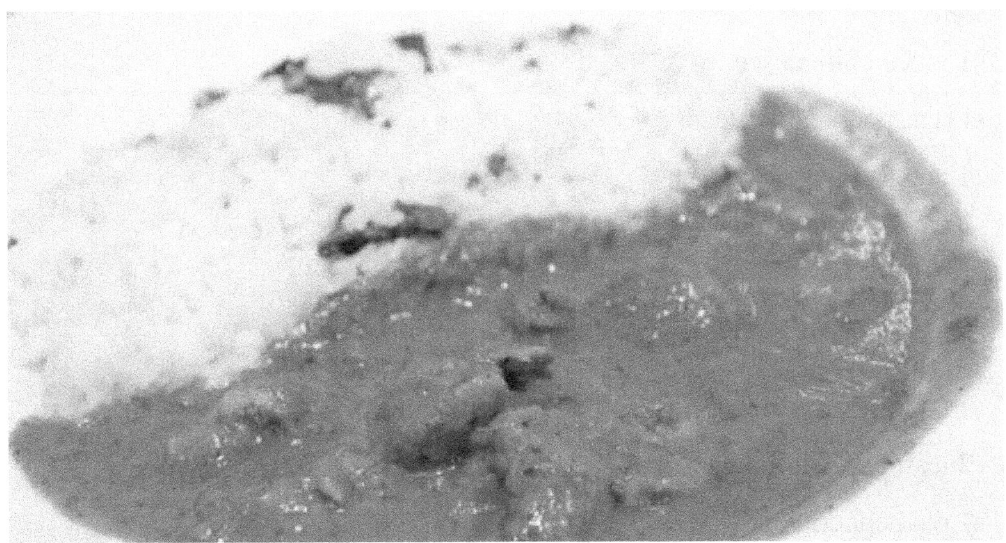

Prep Time: 10 minutes

Cooking Time: 10 minutes

Servings: 4 persons

Quite easy to prepare and absolutely delicious! For a tangy flavor, just squeeze a fresh lemon on top of everything and then sprinkle with some red chili flakes. You can prepare this recipe in the morning and leave it for a complete day. Just re-heat the same before eating.

Ingredients:

- ½ pound lean lamb steak, cubed
- 1 green chili, deseeded & sliced
- ½ teaspoon cumin seeds
- 1 cup fresh baby spinach
- 2 tablespoons mild curry paste
- 1 can coconut cream, approximately 160ml
- 225 g can chopped tomato
- 1 tablespoon coriander, chopped
- 2 teaspoons sunflower oil
- 1 red pepper, deseeded & sliced

Directions:

1. Over moderate heat in a wok; dry-fry the cumin seeds for a couple of seconds and then, add half of the oil; add the lamb and continue to stir-fry until browned, for a minute. Tip the ingredients onto a large plate.

2. Next, add the remaining oil to the wok; stir-fry the chili and pepper until softened, for a few minutes. Stir in the tomatoes, coconut cream and curry paste with half a can of water. Bring it to a simmer, then continue to cook until saucy, for 5 minutes. Add the spinach, lamb and coriander; give the ingredients a good stir and cook for a couple of more minutes, until the spinach has wilted; serve hot with some basmati rice on side and enjoy.

Nutritional Value: kcal: 200, Fat: 15 g, Fiber: 2 g, Protein: 14 g, Carbohydrates: 6 g

Brown Rice Stir-Fry with Coriander Omelette

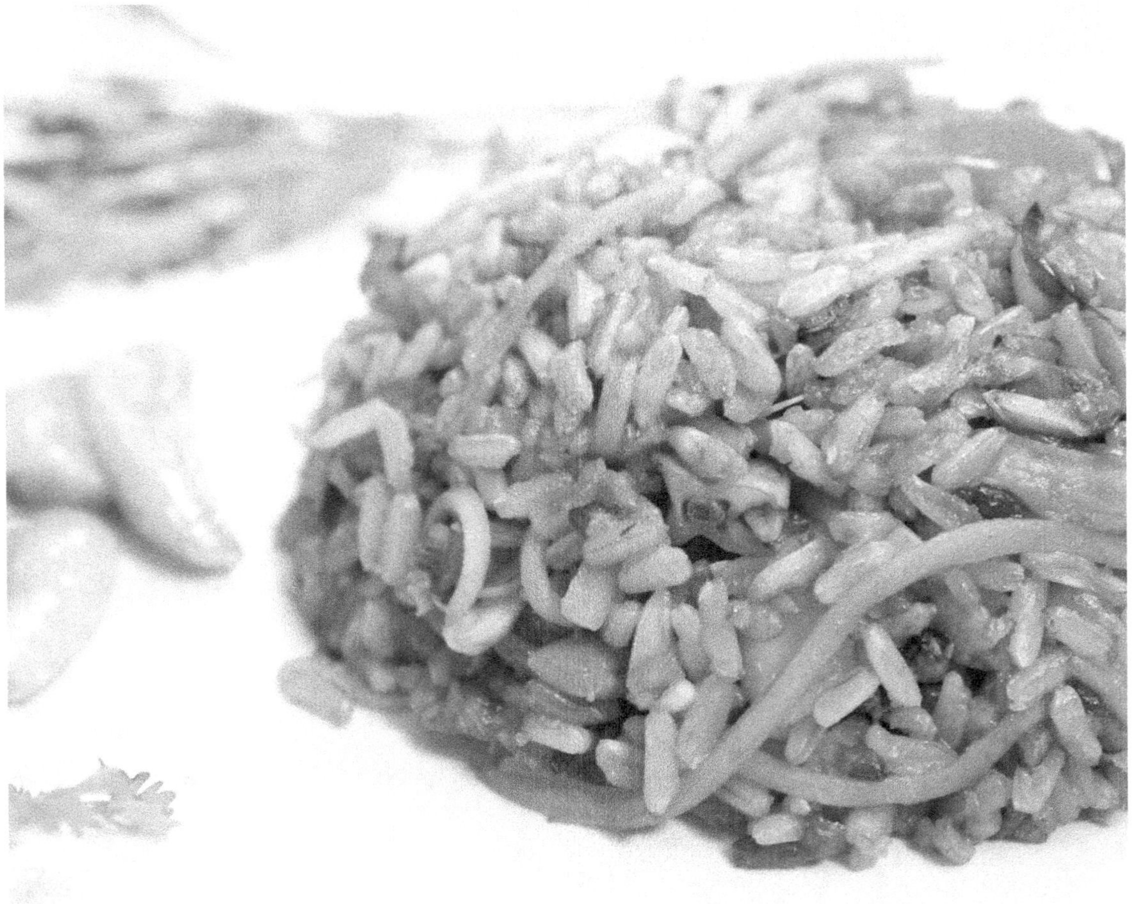

Prep Time: 10 minutes

Cooking Time: 30 minutes

Servings: 4 persons

You can serve this meat-free recipe for your loved ones at a special dinner. You can use fresh chilies along with some ginger and garlic. If you don't have chili jam so you can use kaffir lime leaf sauce and sweet chill.

Ingredients:

- 150g pack shiitake mushroom, sliced
- A bunch of spring onions, finely sliced lengthways
- A piece of ginger, grated (thumb-sized)
- 3 garlic cloves, finely chopped
- 200g brown basmati rice
- 2 carrots, finely sliced into sticks
- 1 red pepper, nicely sliced
- 3 organic eggs, beaten with a splash of skimmed milk
- A small handful coriander, chopped, plus more to serve
- 1 tablespoon sesame seeds, toasted
- 2 teaspoons soy sauce
- 1 teaspoon sesame oil, toasted
- 2 tablespoons chili jam
- 1 tablespoon grape-seed oil

Directions:

1. Prepare the rice per the instructions mentioned on the package. Next, over moderate heat in a wok or large frying pan; heat 2 teaspoons of oil until hot. Once done; carefully add the garlic and ginger; stir-fry for a minute. Tip in the veggies & continue to stir-fry for 3 to 4 minutes, over high heat.

2. In the meantime, combine the eggs with coriander & seasoning in a large-sized mixing bowl. Now, over moderate heat in a small, non-stick frying pan; heat the leftover oil. Then, add the egg; give it a good stir; let cook until almost set, over a gentle heat. Carefully flip & cook the other side for a couple of minutes, until cooked through. Tip onto a clean, large board & then, cut into thin strips.

3. Add the drained cooked rice followed by sesame oil, chili jam and soy sauce to the veggies; continue to mix until heated through. Evenly divide the mixture into separate bowls & top each bowl with the omelette strips, sesame seeds and a few coriander leaves. Serve and enjoy.

Nutritional Value: kcal: 350, Fat: 13 g, Fiber: 4 g, Protein: 15 g, Carbohydrates: 35 g

Beef & Orange Stir-Fry

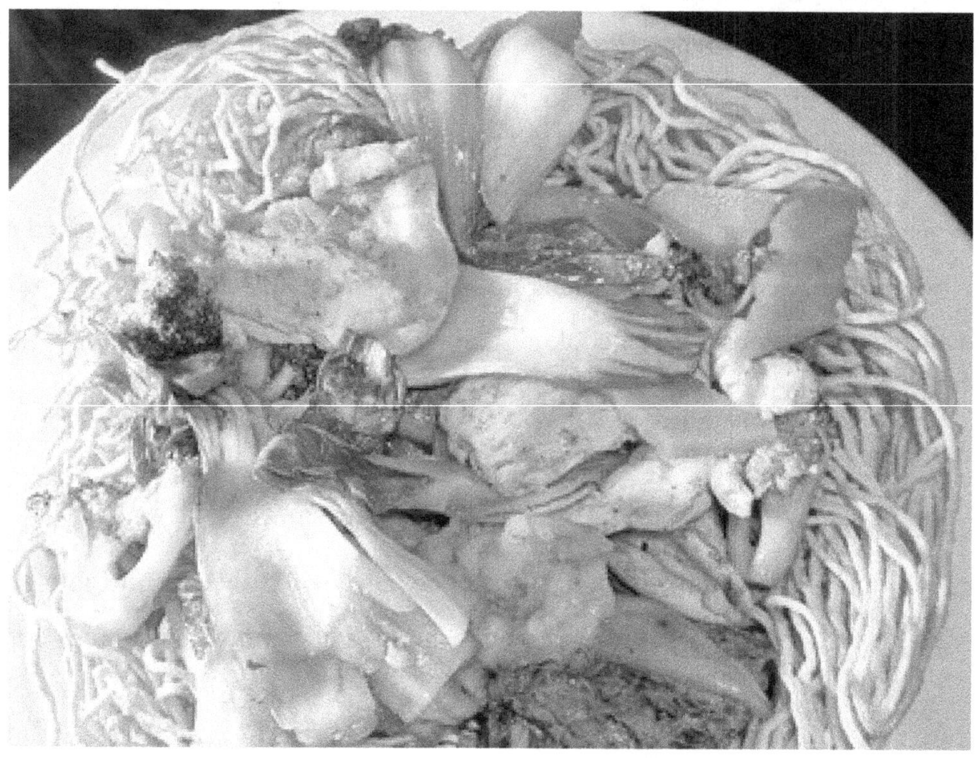

Prep Time: 15 minutes

Cooking Time: 15 minutes

Servings: 3 persons

Your family would fall in love with this recipe. You can serve this recipe with some noodles or steamed cooked rice. Enjoy.

Ingredients:

- 1 pound rump steak, trimmed of any excess fat & cut into very thin strips
- 2 red peppers, deseeded & sliced
- ½ pound Tender stem broccoli or purple sprouting
- 2 teaspoons corn flour
- A piece of ginger, peeled & cut into matchsticks (thumb-sized)
- 4 spring onions, halved & sliced lengthways
- 1 red chili, deseeded & thinly sliced
- 4 garlic cloves, finely chopped
- 1½ tablespoons clear honey
- 2 oranges, 1 cut into segments & 1 juiced
- 1 tablespoon dark soy sauce
- 4 teaspoons groundnut oil
- 1 tablespoon rice vinegar

Directions:

1. Boil or steam the broccoli until tender, for 3 to 4 minutes. Drain & run the pieces under cold running tap water.

2. Next, over moderate heat in a large frying pan or non-stick wok; heat 2 teaspoons of oil until hot. In the meantime; toss the beef strips into the corn flour. When the oil turns hot, carefully add the beef & fry until turn brown, for a minute or two; put the pieces to one side.

3. Next, heat the leftover oil in the pan until hot and then toss in the peppers; fry for a minute then, add the garlic, ginger, 3 spring onions and chili; cook for a minute more (ensure that you don't burn the garlic). Add the honey, orange juice, soy and rice vinegar; let cook for a couple of minutes and then, stir in the beef, broccoli & orange segments. Continue to cook until heated through then, sprinkle with the leftover spring onion. Serve immediately & enjoy.

Nutritional Value: kcal: 330, Fat: 11 g, Fiber: 6 g, Protein: 34 g, Carbohydrates: 25 g

Soup & Salad

Curried Squash, Lentil & Coconut Soup

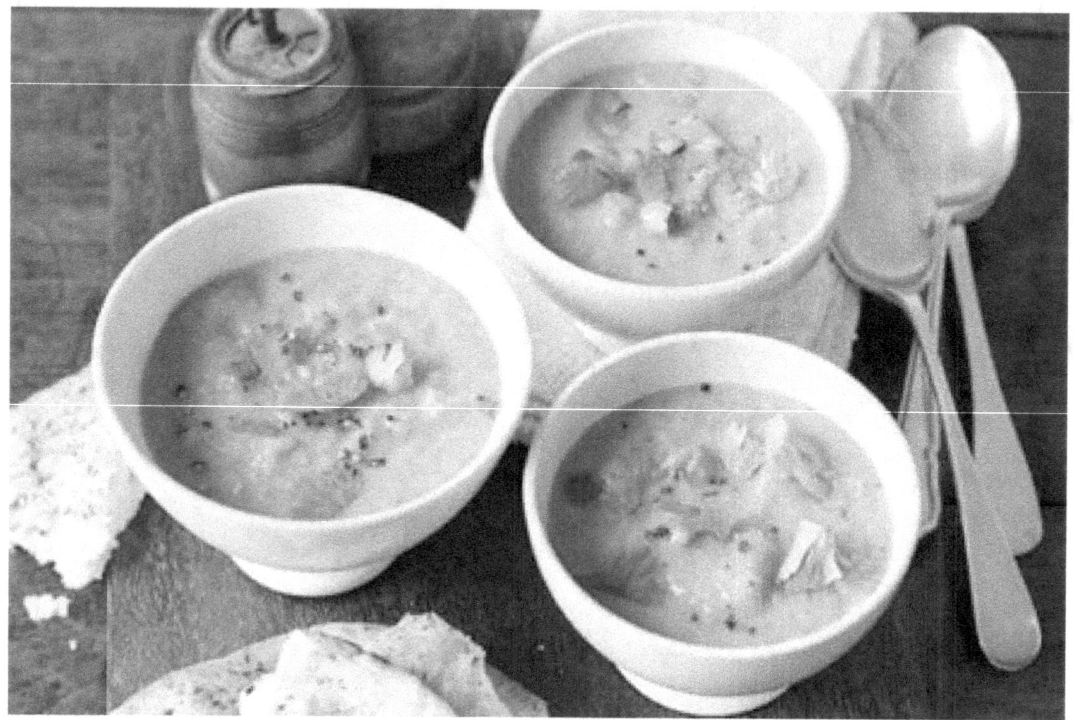

Prep Time: 10 minutes

Cooking Time: 30 minutes

Servings: 6 persons

Just add a couple of dashes of sriracha to increase the taste of this soup and serve it to the guests with some roughly chopped coriander and naan bread.

Ingredients:

- 1 butternut squash, peeled, deseeded & diced
- ¼ pound red lentil
- 1 can coconut milk, reduced-fat
- ½ pound carrot, diced
- 1 tablespoon olive oil
- 5 cups vegetable stock, low-sodium
- 1 tablespoon curry powder containing turmeric

Directions:

1. Over moderate heat in a large saucepan; heat the oil until hot and then, add the carrots and squash, sizzle for a minute and then, stir in the curry powder; continue to cook for a minute.

2. Add the lentils followed by the coconut milk and vegetable stock; give the ingredients a good stir until evenly mixed. Bring the mixture to a boil. Once done; decrease the heat & let simmer until tender, for 15 to 20 minutes.

3. Blitz in a food processor or in a hand blender until you get your desired smoothness. Season & serve immediately.

Nutritional Value: kcal: 170, Fat: 7 g, Fiber: 4 g, Protein: 7 g, Carbohydrates: 22 g

Caramelized Onion & Barley Soup with Cheese Croutons

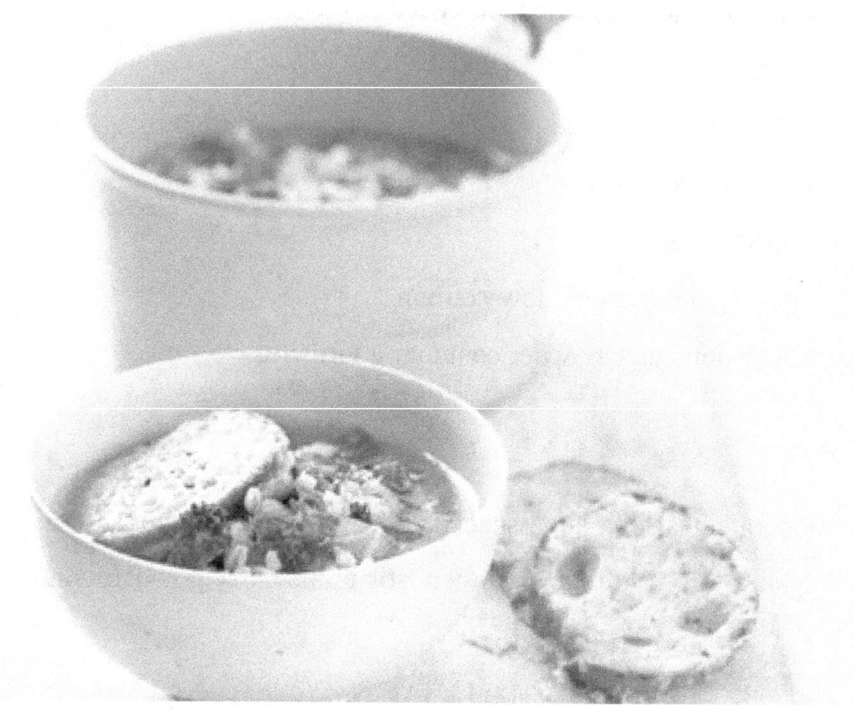

Prep Time: 10 minutes

Cooking Time: 40 minutes

Servings: 2 persons

I was looking for a barley recipe with something different, so I come up with this. This soup turned out to be so delicious that my family asked me to prepare this soup again. Just loved it!

Ingredients:

- 2 medium onions, sliced thinly
- 4 tablespoons gruyère cheese, grated
- 6 thyme sprigs, fresh, chopped
- 4 ½ cups vegetable stock
- 2 cloves garlic, thinly sliced
- ½ cup kale or cavolo nero, discard any thick stalks & slice the leaves
- 2 tablespoons barley
- 4 slices baguette, toasted
- 1 tablespoon olive oil
- A good pinch of sugar

Directions:

1. Over moderate heat in a large saucepan; heat the oil until hot and then add the garlic followed by onions, thyme, a good pinch of salt and sugar. Cook until turn golden in color, for 15 to 20 minutes. Add the stock; give the ingredients a good stir and let simmer for 10 more minutes.

2. Fill a separate large saucepan with lightly salted water, bring it to a boil. Once done add & cook the barley for 12 to 15 minutes. During the last three minutes of cooking; don't forget to add the kale or cavolo nero. Drain & rinse under cold running tap water. Then, add to the soup. Continue to cook until heated through.

3. Now, heat up your grill. Top the toasted bread with cheese; place under the grill and cook for a minute or two, until melted and bubbly. Serve the soup in two large bowls with some cheesy croutons on top.

Nutritional Value: kcal: 430, Fat: 15 g, Fiber: 6 g, Protein: 16 g, Carbohydrates: 40 g

Delicious Summer Soup

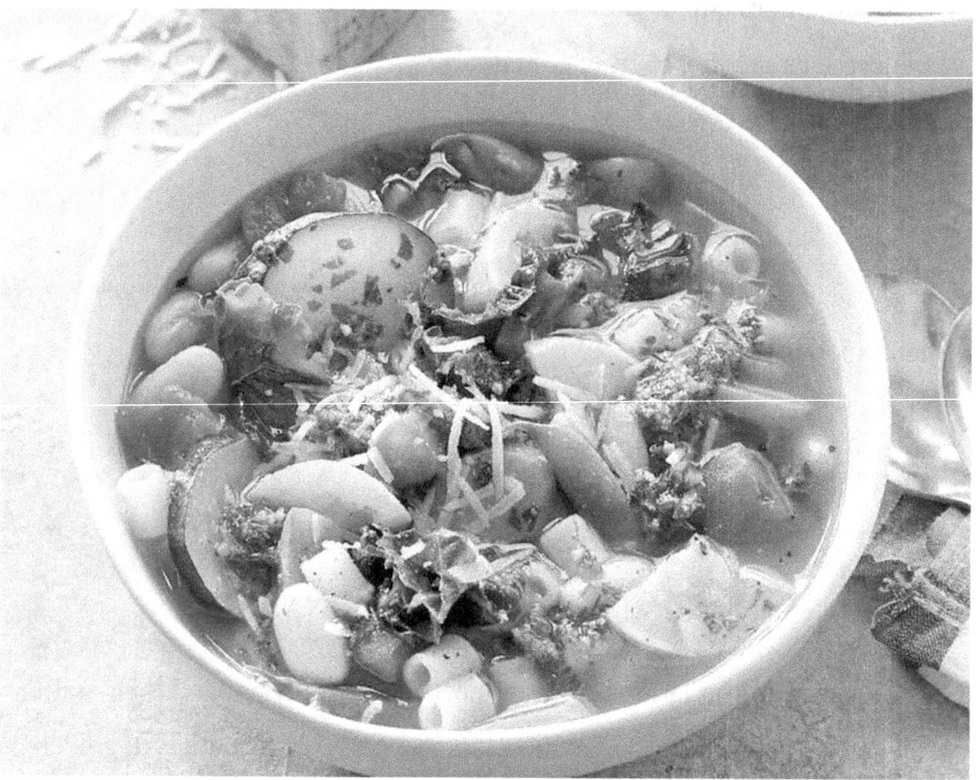

Prep Time: 20 minutes

Cooking Time: 20 minutes

Servings: 4 persons

When it comes to soup, I expect it to be very healthy and super delicious. I have personally prepared it so many times, and each time, it was a hit. If you are looking for a thick version of the soup, then you must try leeks than spring onions.

Ingredients:

- 2 rounded tablespoons Greek yogurt, plus more for serving
- ½ pound pea, fresh or frozen, podded
- 3 courgettes, chopped
- A bunch of spring onions, chopped
- 6 cups hot vegetable stock
- A large handful of fresh mint
- 85g bag trimmed watercress
- Splash of olive oil/knob of butter

Directions:

1. Over moderate heat in a large pan; heat the oil or butter. Once done; carefully add the spring onions followed by the courgettes; give the ingredients a good stir. Cover & cook for a couple of minutes. Add the stock and peas. Then, bring it to a boil, over moderate heat. Cover & let simmer for a couple of more minutes, then remove from the heat; give it a good stir and then add the mint and watercress; continue to stir until wilted.

2. Add the hot soup in a food processor & purée; adding the yogurt in the second batch. Pour the soup into the pan again and then add some seasoning to taste. Serve hot drizzled with more of yogurt. Enjoy.

Nutritional Value: kcal: 100, Fat: 4 g, Fiber: 4 g, Protein: 8 g, Carbohydrates: 9 g

Beef Goulash Soup

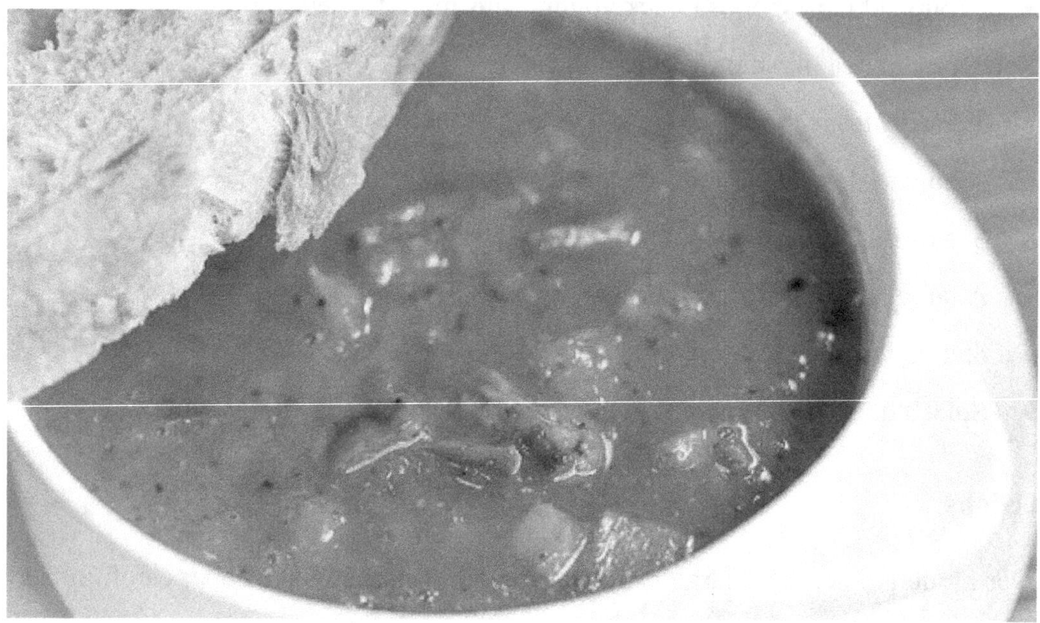

Prep Time: 10 minutes

Cooking Time: 1 hour & 20 minutes

Servings: 3 persons

If you are actually looking for a beef soup recipe which is healthy for your tummy, then you must try this one. With this, you can give your loved ones more protein than they actually need. For more heat, you can add more paprika and hot chili pepper.

Ingredients:

- 1 onion, preferably large-sized, halved & sliced
- 1 medium sweet potato, peeled & diced
- 3 cloves garlic, sliced
- 1 teaspoon caraway seeds
- ½ pound stewing beef, extra lean, diced finely
- 1 can tomatoes, chopped (approximately 1 pound)
- 2 teaspoons smoked paprika
- 1 green pepper, remove the seeds, diced
- 4 cups beef stock
- 1 tablespoon grape seed oil

For Topping:

- A good handful of fresh parsley, chopped
- 1 pot good quality yogurt (approximately 150 g)

Directions:

1. Over moderate heat in a large pan; heat the oil until hot. Once done, carefully add the garlic and onion; stir-fry until changes its color, for 3 to 5 minutes. Add the beef; give the ingredients a good stir and increase the heat; continue to fry until turn brown, stirring frequently.

2. Add the paprika and caraway, stir well and then add the tomatoes followed by the stock. Cover & gently cook for 25 to 30 minutes.

3. Add the green pepper and sweet potato; give the ingredients a good stir until nicely mixed. Cover & cook until tender, for 20 minutes more. Let cool down a bit; serve immediately; topped with some fresh yogurt & fresh parsley.

Nutritional Value: kcal: 345, Fat: 12 g, Fiber: 7 g, Protein: 25 g, Carbohydrates: 28 g

Shaved Fennel, Courgette & Orange Salad

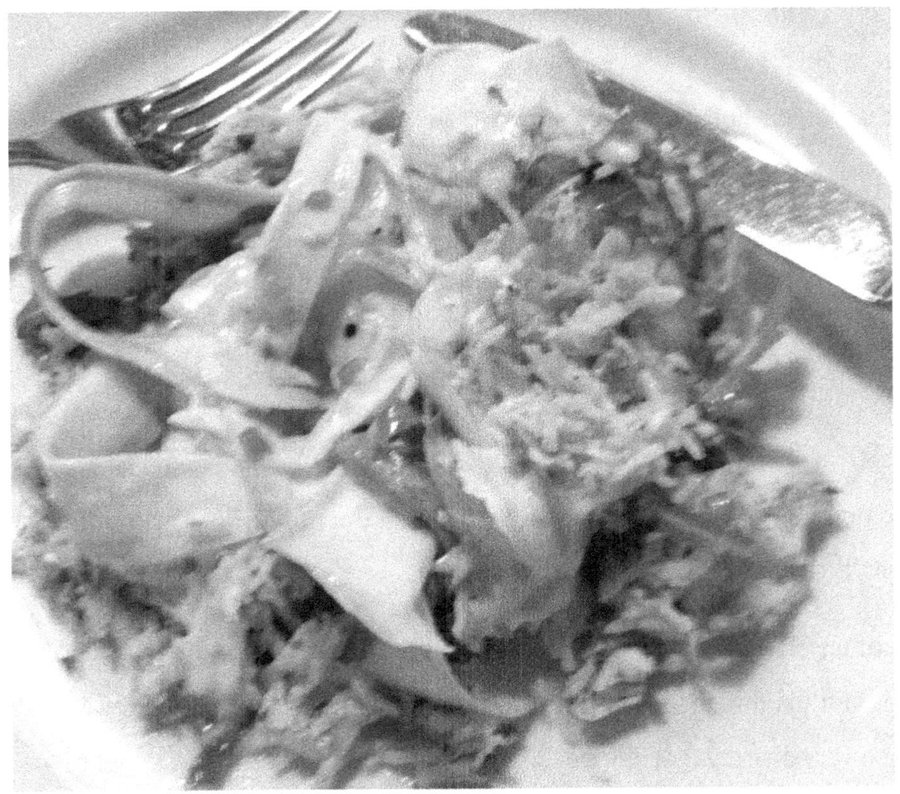

Prep Time: 10 minutes

Cooking Time: 15 minutes

Servings: 4 persons

This is one of the best salad recipes that I have ever prepared for my family. Fresh &crisp, this salad includes zesty orange with crunchy courgette and tangy fennel. Don't forget to dress the salad at during the last minute. Serve and enjoy.

Ingredients:

- 2 small fennel bulbs
- 1 orange
- 2 teaspoons sherry vinegar
- 1 fresh lettuce, leaves separated & washed
- 2 small courgettes (green or yellow)
- Juice of ½ a lemon, freshly squeezed
- 4 tablespoons olive oil

Directions:

1. Peel the orange using a serrated knife; removing the pith. Slice the orange; cutting each slice into half (don't forget to reserve any juice).

2. Get rid of any tough leaves from fennel. Halve; cut the cores out and then slice using a sharp mandolin (as thin as possible); trimming the ends from the courgettes and shave off long using a very sharp vegetable peeler and then cut it into thin slices; get rid of any seedy & watery centers.

3. Combine the kept-aside orange juice with olive oil and sherry vinegar. Season well; add the lemon juice; mix well. Just before you serve the dish, don't forget to mix the courgette, fennel, orange slices and lettuce leaves with the prepared dressing.

Nutritional Value: kcal: 170, Fat: 12 g, Fiber: 4 g, Protein: 4 g, Carbohydrates: 10 g

Conclusion

Thank you again for downloading this e-book.

If you are really looking for healthy immune, then you must go for natural foods and eliminate processed foods from your diet.

The advantage of healthy immune is just not only weight loss, but it also goes beyond your expectations.

Remember that a healthy immune system would keep you energized throughout the day, your skin would glow, your eyes would look more alert and brighter, and you wouldn't catch infections easily.

What are you still waiting for? If you haven't downloaded this e-book till yet, then do it now and forget about the health of your loved ones. This e-book would help you and your family maintain healthy immune system.

About the Author

Born in New Germantown, Pennsylvania, Stephanie Sharp received a Masters degree from Penn State in English Literature. Driven by her passion to create culinary masterpieces, she applied and was accepted to The International Culinary School of the Art Institute where she excelled in French cuisine. She has married her cooking skills with an aptitude for business by opening her own small cooking school where she teaches students of all ages.

Stephanie's talents extend to being an author as well and she has written over 400 e-books on the art of cooking and baking that include her most popular recipes.

Sharp has been fortunate enough to raise a family near her hometown in Pennsylvania where she, her husband and children live in a beautiful rustic house on an extensive piece of land. Her other passion is taking care of the furry members of her family which include 3 cats, 2 dogs and a potbelly pig named Wilbur.

Watch for more amazing books by Stephanie Sharp coming out in the next few months.

Author's Afterthoughts

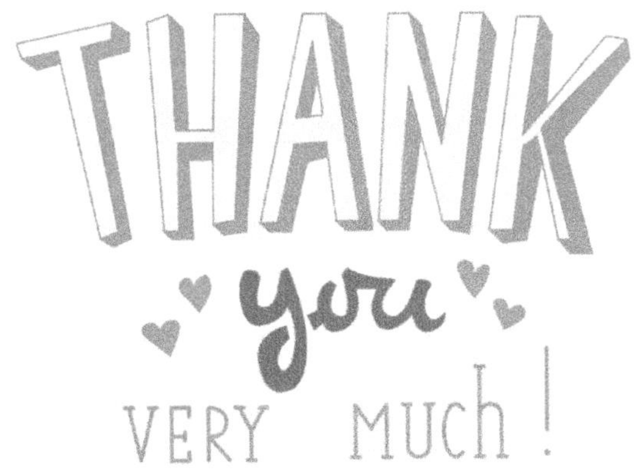

I am truly grateful to you for taking the time to read my book. I cherish all of my readers! Thanks ever so much to each of my cherished readers for investing the time to read this book!

With so many options available to you, your choice to buy my book is an honour, so my heartfelt thanks at reading it from beginning to end!

I value your feedback, so please take a moment to submit an honest and open review on Amazon so I can get valuable insight into my readers' opinions and others can benefit from your experience.

Thank you for taking the time to review!

Stephanie Sharp